Golwalla's
ELECTROCARDIOGRAPHY
For Medical Students and General Practitioners

Golwalla's
ELECTROCARDIOGRAPHY
For Medical Students and General Practitioners

FIFTEENTH EDITION

Revised and Edited by

Sharukh A Golwalla
MD (Med) DM (Card)
Visiting Cardiologist
Breach Candy Hospital, Jaslok Hospital
HN Reliance Foundation Hospital
Mumbai, Maharashtra, India

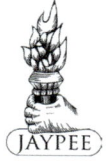

JAYPEE BROTHERS MEDICAL PUBLISHERS
The Health Sciences Publisher
New Delhi | London

Jaypee Brothers Medical Publishers (P) Ltd

Headquarters
EMCA House
23/23-B, Ansari Road, Daryaganj
New Delhi 110 002, India
Landline: +91-11-23272143, +91-11-23272703
+91-11-23282021, +91-11-23245672
E-mail: jaypee@jaypeebrothers.com

Corporate Office
Jaypee Brothers Medical Publishers (P) Ltd.
4838/24, Ansari Road, Daryaganj
New Delhi 110 002, India
Phone: +91-11-43574357
Fax: +91-11-43574314
E-mail: jaypee@jaypeebrothers.com

Overseas Office
JP Medical Ltd.
83, Victoria Street, London
SW1H 0HW (UK)
Phone: +44-20 3170 8910
Fax: +44(0)20 3008 6180
E-mail: info@jpmedpub.com

Website: www.jaypeebrothers.com
Website: www.jaypeedigital.com

© 2022, Jaypee Brothers Medical Publishers

The views and opinions expressed in this book are solely those of the original contributor(s)/author(s) and do not necessarily represent those of editor(s) of the book.

All rights reserved by the author. No part of this publication may be reproduced, stored or transmitted in any form or by any means, electronic, mechanical, photocopying, recording or otherwise, without the prior permission in writing of the publishers.

All brand names and product names used in this book are trade names, service marks, trademarks or registered trademarks of their respective owners. The publisher is not associated with any product or vendor mentioned in this book.

Medical knowledge and practice change constantly. This book is designed to provide accurate, authoritative information about the subject matter in question. However, readers are advised to check the most current information available on procedures included and check information from the manufacturer of each product to be administered, to verify the recommended dose, formula, method and duration of administration, adverse effects and contraindications. It is the responsibility of the practitioner to take all appropriate safety precautions. Neither the publisher nor the author(s)/editor(s) assume any liability for any injury and/or damage to persons or property arising from or related to use of material in this book.

This book is sold on the understanding that the publisher is not engaged in providing professional medical services. If such advice or services are required, the services of a competent medical professional should be sought.

Every effort has been made where necessary to contact holders of copyright to obtain permission to reproduce copyright material. If any have been inadvertently overlooked, the publisher will be pleased to make the necessary arrangements at the first opportunity.

Inquiries for bulk sales may be solicited at: jaypee@jaypeebrothers.com

Golwalla's Electrocardiography for Medical Students and General Practitioners

First Edition: 1955

Fifteenth Edition: **2022**

ISBN 978-93-5465-492-3

Printed at: Sterling Graphics Pvt. Ltd. India.

PREFACE

With the passing away of the original author, this simplified book of *Electrocardiography for Medical Students and General Practitioners* continues to fulfill its primary aim of learning basic electrocardiography (ECG). Many new ECG tracings and some revised texts make the book easier to digest. M/s Jaypee Brothers Medical Publishers (P) Ltd, New Delhi, India have kindly taken over the responsibility of distributing this edition all over the country, for which I am very grateful.

Sharukh A Golwalla

October 2021

CONTENTS

1. **Introduction**   1
   - ¤ Basic Principles   1
   - ¤ Basic Electrophysiology   1
   - ¤ Normal Sequence of Cardiac Depolarization and Repolarization   2
   - ¤ ECG Registration—Types of Leads   4
     - Bipolar Limb Leads or Standard Leads   4
     - Unipolar Leads   5
2. **The Normal Electrocardiogram**   9
   - ¤ Normal Electrocardiographic Complex   9
   - ¤ Normal Patterns and Variations of the Electrocardiogram   11
   - ¤ Electrocardiographic Position of the Heart   13
     - Rotation on Anteroposterior Axis   13
     - Rotation on Longitudinal Axis   14
3. **Method of Analysis of the Electrocardiogram**   15
   - ¤ Rate   16
   - ¤ Rhythm   18
     - Sinus Rhythm   18
     - Atrial Rhythms   20
     - Junctional (Nodal) Rhythm   24
     - Ventricular Rhythms   25
     - Atrioventricular Conduction Variations   27
     - Unusual Complexes or Beats   30
   - ¤ Voltage   34
   - ¤ Electrical Axis   35
     - Procedure for Determining the Electrical Axis   36
   - ¤ P Wave Abnormalities   39
     - Duration and Amplitude: Chamber Enlargement   39
     - Absent (Unidentifiable) P waves   40
     - Inverted P Waves   41
     - Changing Shape   43
   - ¤ PR Interval Abnormalities   43
     - Prolonged   43
     - Shortened   43
     - Varying   43

- ¤ Q Wave Abnormalities   44
  - Pathological Q Wave   44
- ¤ QRS Complex Abnormalities   44
  - Duration and Amplitude   44
- ¤ ST Segment Abnormalities   54
  - Depressed   54
  - Elevated   55
- ¤ T Wave Abnormalities   60
  - Increased Amplitude   60
  - Low or Flat   61
  - Inverted   61
- ¤ QT Interval Abnormalities   62
  - Prolonged   62
  - Shortened   62
- ¤ U Wave Abnormalities   63
- ¤ J wave   63

4. Ischemic Heart Disease   65

- ¤ Myocardial Infarction   65
  - ECG Changes in ST Segment Elevation MI   65
  - ECG Changes in Non-ST Segment Elevation MI   69
- ¤ Myocardial Ischemia without infarction   72
  - ECG at Rest   72
  - ECG During Anginal Attack   72
  - No Pain   73
  - Chest Pain   73
  - Prinzmetal's (Variant) Angina   73
  - The Brugada Syndrome   74

CHAPTER 1

Introduction

■ BASIC PRINCIPLES

When the heart contracts, electric currents are produced and distributed throughout the body to the skin. Two electrodes can be applied to any two parts of the body to lead the heart current to a recording galvanometer. The graphic representation of these electric currents is called an electrocardiogram.

■ BASIC ELECTROPHYSIOLOGY

The changes in the electrical potential with each heart beat can be understood by considering the electrical behavior of a single cell. The surface of the resting cell will be electrically positive compared with the interior of the cell which is electrically negative. A cell in this condition is said to be in the 'polarized' state **(Fig. 1A)** and the exterior and interior of the cell can be compared to the two poles of a battery. When the cell is stimulated, the positive ions migrate into the cell and the negative ions migrate out of the cell. With this reversal of polarity, the cell is said to be 'depolarized' **(Fig. 1B)**. When the effect of excitation has passed off and the cell has returned to its former resting state, the positive charge outside and negative charge inside are restored, the cell is 'repolarized' **(Fig. 1C)**.

When an excitatory (depolarization) process flows towards a unipolar electrode, the galvanometer will record a positive or upward deflection, and when it flows away from the electrode, a negative or downward deflection **(Fig. 2)**:

Thus, the excitation and subsequent recovery of the muscle strip have given rise to two electrical currents or deflections of opposite directions. The currents of repolarization (during recovery) are weaker and extend over a longer period of time than those of depolarization (during excitation). Applying this to the electrical changes produced

Introduction

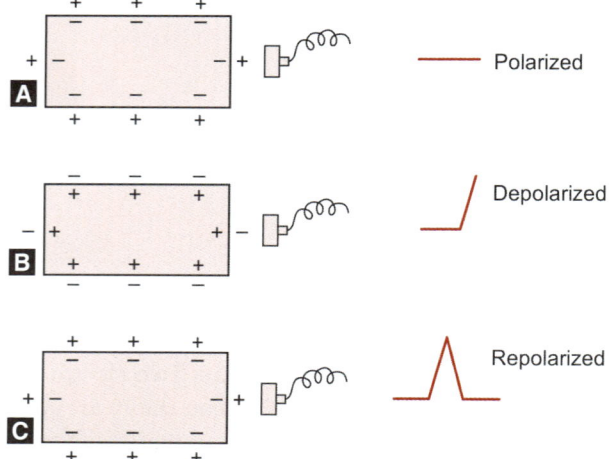

Figs. 1A to C: Illustrates: (A) Polarized; (B) Depolarized; and (C) Repolarized cell.

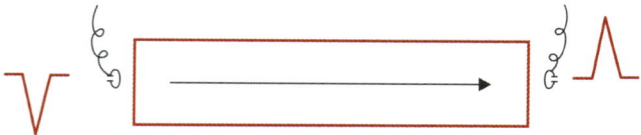

Fig. 2: Illustrates the electrical behavior of a single cell or strip of muscle, indicated by a rectangle from the two ends of which the potentials are led off to a galvanometer.

by the heart beats, the same fundamental principle holds but with some modifications. This is because the heart consists of a multitude of intercommunicating muscle fibers and has four chambers which are activated in sequence more complicated than the simple spread of excitation through a muscle strip.

■ NORMAL SEQUENCE OF CARDIAC DEPOLARIZATION AND REPOLARIZATION

The normal process of activation begins in the sinoatrial (SA) node and spreads through the atria in a lateral and downward direction (**Fig. 3,** arrow 1). Since the atria are thin-walled structures, little electrical activity results from their depolarization—**P wave**. An electrode placed on the left side of the body will record an upright P wave, on the right side a negative P wave.

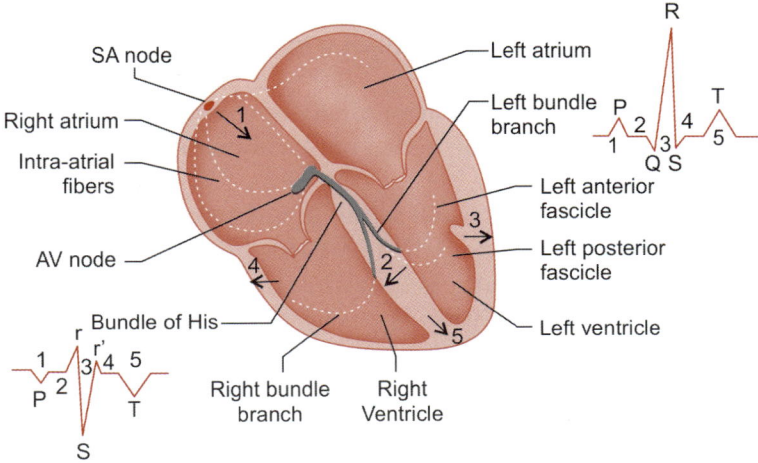

Fig. 3: Sequence of electrical activation in the heart.

The wave of depolarization then activates the atrioventricular (AV) node where there is a 1/10 second delay to allow the ventricles to fill prior to ventricular systole. During this time, electrical activity moves very slowly through the AV node and then into the ventricles through the proximal portion of the ventricular conducting system, the bundle of His and the bundle branches, the septum being activated from, left to right. All these structures are so small that electrical activity within them is not detected and on the ECG no movement of the base line is seen—the isoelectric **PR interval.**

Activation spreads into the main mass of ventricular muscle from the subendocardial region outwards. Electrocardiographically the ventricles are made up of three muscle groups—right ventricle (RV), interventricular septum (which behaves as a left ventricular structure) and the left ventricle (LV). The first portion of ventricular depolarization in the ECG results from septal depolarization from left to right (**Fig. 3,** arrow 2). Since the septum is smaller than the bulk of the myocardium, this initial deflection is relatively small—**q wave.**

The depolarization then spreads outwards simultaneously through the free ventricular walls from endocardial to epicardial surface (**Fig. 3,** arrow 3). The thick left ventricular electrical force counteracts the smaller right ventricular force. A large upright deflection **R** is thus produced in a left-sided electrode. Sometimes, late activation of an upper part of the right ventricle (**Fig. 3,** arrow 4) produces a late negative deflection S. The QRS pattern recorded by a left-sided electrode is mirrored by an rsr' pattern in an electrode on the right side of the chest **(Fig. 3)**.

After the ventricle has been totally depolarized, there is no electrical activity for a brief period until repolarization begins—**ST segment.**

Repolarization, that is the return of myocardial cells to their resulting negative potential then proceeds from endocardium to epicardium. Ventricular repolarization produces—**T** wave. The recovery process **(Fig. 3,** arrow 5) is much slower than the activation and the—T wave is generally a broad deflection in a similar direction as a rule to the main wave of the QRS complex (upright in left-sided electrodes).

After the conclusion of repolarization, there is again a period of electrical inactivity and the base line of the ECG remains isoelectric until the next impulse originates producing the next series of P-QRS-T complexes.

ECG REGISTRATION—TYPES OF LEADS

The term lead is used to denote the connection of the galvanometer by wires to the electrodes and also for the actual tracing obtained. Although two electrodes can be attached to any part of the body to lead the heart current to the galvanometer, it is customary to make use of the forearms, the left leg and the precordium.

Each chamber of the heart produces a characteristic electrocardiographic pattern. Since the electrical potentials over the various areas of the heart differ, the recorded tracings from each limb vary accordingly.

1. Bipolar Limb Leads or Standard Leads

Here two electrodes are placed on two extremities and both record simultaneously the particular electrical pattern of the heart facing these extremities **(Fig. 4)**.

Lead 1: Records the potential between the left arm electrode (positive pole) and right arm electrode. Thus when an electric current moves through the heart from right arm to left arm a positive deflection is recorded in lead I.

Introduction

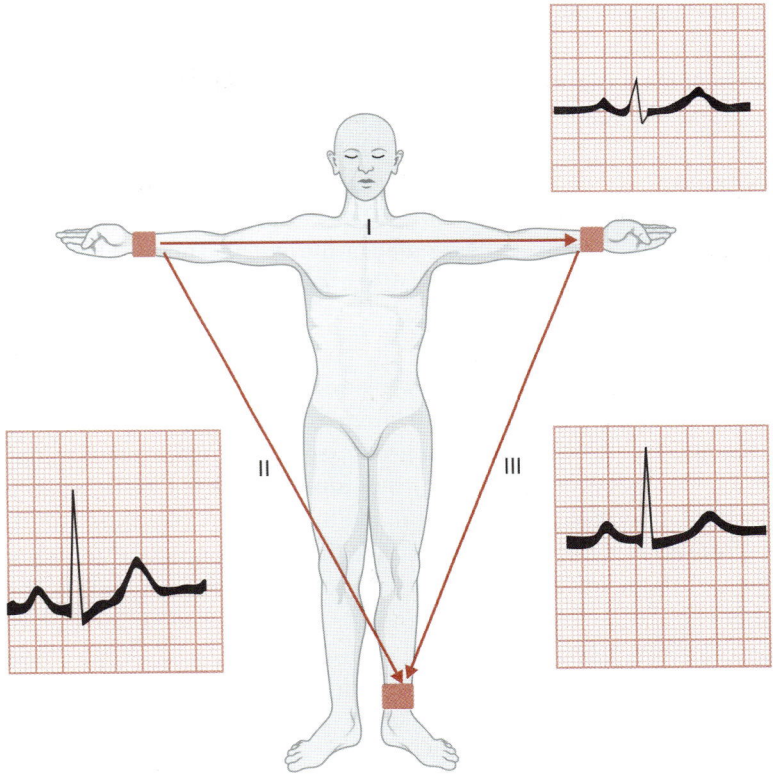

Fig. 4: Limb leads.

Lead II: Left leg (positive pole) and right arm. An electric current moving from the right arm diagonally downward to the left leg causes an upward deflection in lead II.

Lead III: Positive pole is at left leg and negative pole at left arm. A current flowing from left arm to left leg records a positive deflection in lead III.

Although electrodes are attached to both legs, the right leg electrode is used as spare or ground since recordings obtained from the other leg are identical.

2. Unipolar Leads

Each standard limb lead, it will be obvious, is in reality a combination of two tracings. It would be however an advantage to obtain a final pattern of the electrocardiogram which would represent the unaltered potential of one area of the heart. This can be achieved with the unipolar technique.

Unipolar leads are obtained by placing one electrode (exploring electrode) in close proximity to the heart, while the other indifferent electrode is far removed from it so that its potential is more or less reduced to zero.

All unipolar leads are designated by the letter V. There are two types of unipolar leads — unipolar limb leads and unipolar chest leads.

Unipolar Limb Leads

These are registered by a recording system in which one electrode is placed in turn, over one of the three extremities used in recording standard leads, while the other is connected to the central terminal. With this technique however, the amplitude of the deflections is so small that their interpretation is difficult. The amplitude can be increased by 50% if the exploring electrode is attached to either the right arm, left arm, or left leg and connected to one pole of the galvanometer, whilst the other pole is connected to an indifferent lead point—a central terminal connecting the remaining three extremities not being explored. They are therefore called augmented limb or extremity leads and the letter 'a' is used as prefix to denote augmentation.

From **Figure 5,** it will be seen that the electrical picture present at any particular extremity covers a variable surface of the heart. Since the electrical potentials over various areas of the heart differ, the recorded patterns from each limb will also vary.

Lead aVR: The electrode of the right forearm, conveys the electrical picture of the heart as it presents itself at the right shoulder and reflects the potential variations of the atrial and ventricular cavities.

Lead aVL: Conveys the electrical potentials from the left lateral cardiac wall.

Lead aVF: Which corresponds to the center of the left lower limb with the trunk, reflects the potential of the diaphragmatic or inferior surface of the heart.

The basic information obtained from these leads is the same as bipolar limb leads. The six limb leads provide a round the clock view of cardiac electrical activity in the *frontal* plane of the body.

Introduction

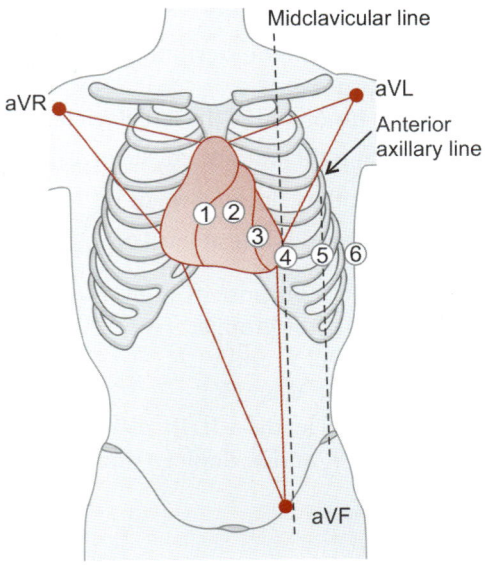

Fig. 5: Augmented limb leads, and precordial leads V_1–V_6. Each augmented limb lead is visualized as a solid cone projecting on to the surface of the heart.

Unipolar Precordial or Chest Leads (Fig. 5)

Direct leads from the various points on the heart itself present the most detailed information regarding the spread of the excitation wave through the heart and abnormalities thereof. The best substitute for such direct leads is precordial leads with the exploring electrode placed on the skin over the part of the heart which it is desired to study. A series of six positions across the precordium (leads V_1 to V_6) have been chosen for standard recording giving a round the clock view of the *horizontal plane* of the heart **(Fig. 5)**:

V_1 : 4th intercostal space right sternal border.
V_2 : 4th intercostal space left sternal border.
V_3 : Midway between V_2 and V_4.
V_4 : 5th intercostal space in midclavicular line.
V_5 : 5th intercostal space in anterior axillary line
V_6 : Midaxillary line at level of V_4.

Additional leads sometimes recorded are:

Ve	:	Inferior border of the sternum, slightly to the left of the ensiform process.
VSc	:	Below the inner end of the left clavicle.
V_3R, V_4R	:	Position on right anterior chest corresponding to V_3, V_4.
V_7	:	Posterior axillary line at level of V_4.
V_8	:	Posterior scapular line at level of V_4.

Lead Classification, for the purpose of analysis the 12 leads that are usually recorded fall into three groups:
1. Left-sided leads — I, aVL, V_5 and V_6.
2. Right-sided leads — aVR, V_1 and V_2.
3. Inferior (diaphragmatic) leads — II, III, aVF

Mid-precordial leads V_3 and V_4 depict a transition between right- and left-sided patterns.

CHAPTER 2

The Normal Electrocardiogram

■ NORMAL ELECTROCARDIOGRAPHIC COMPLEX (FIGURE 6)

- *P wave:* Due to spread of stimulus through the atria. It is usually an upright small round deflection.
- *QRS complex:* Due to electrical stimulation (contraction) of the ventricles. *Q wave* — An initial downward deflection of QRS complex. *R wave* — An initial upward deflection, or an upward

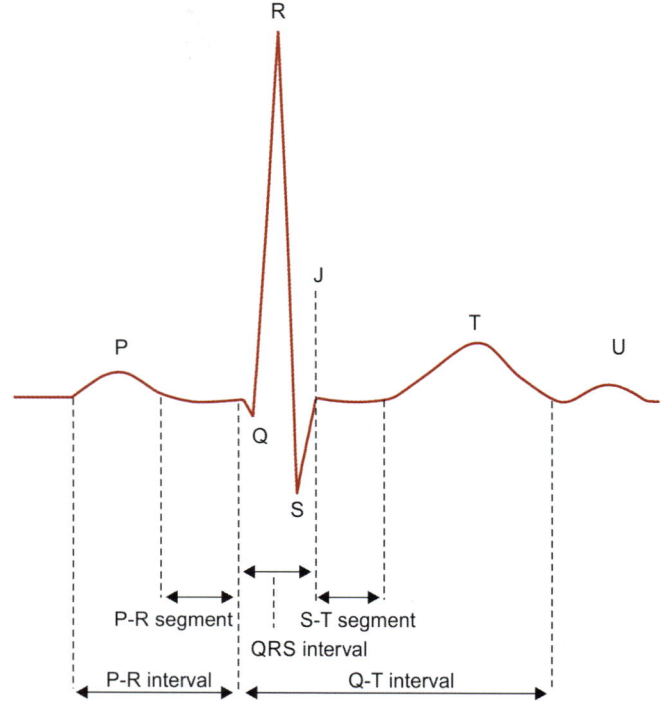

Fig. 6: Diagram of normal electrocardiographic complex.

deflection which is preceded by a Q wave. *S wave* — A downward deflection following R.
- *R' wave:* A second upward deflection after an R wave.
- *S' wave:* A second downward deflection after R'.
- If there is only one deflection and it is downward, it is called QS.
- *ST segment:* The base line between S and T waves.
- *T wave:* A somewhat broad deflection in a similar direction as a rule to the main wave of the QRS complex.

- *Isoelectric line:* The point at which ST segment joins the QRS complex is termed junction J. It is often in the base line or isoelectric level or the zero position of the record in normal persons.
- *U wave:* A small upright rounded deflection following the T wave.

All upward deflections are called positive. All downward deflections are termed negative. A Q or S wave is never directed upward, and an R wave can never be directed downward. A Q wave must always be situated in front of the R and an S wave must always follow the R. Smaller amplitude waves are termed q, r and s waves **(Fig. 7)**.

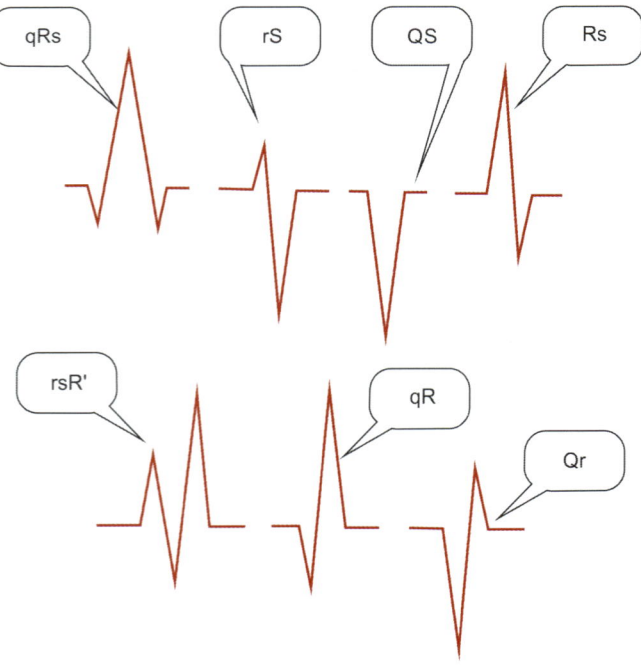

Fig. 7: Various QRS complexes.

Normal Time Intervals. These are subject to biological variability, and factors such as age, sex and heart rate must be considered when interpreting these measurements.

PR interval: It is measured from the beginning of the P wave to the beginning of the QRS complex. It represents the atrioventricular conduction time and varies from 0.12 to 0.2 seconds, average 0.16 second. It tends to be shorter with more rapid rates and longer with slower rates.

QRS interval: It is measured from the beginning of the Q wave to the end of the S wave indicates the time it takes for the impulse to spread through the two ventricles and reflects the integrity of the conducting system. The duration of QRS should be measured in the lead showing the longest interval. The normal value lies between 0.06–0.10 seconds. A value greater than 0.10 seconds is abnormal and implies an intraventricular conduction disorder.

QT interval: It represents the total electrical activity of the ventricles. It is measured from the onset of Q wave to the end of the T wave. QT interval is markedly affected by the heart rate; it shortens as the heart rate rises. A useful rule of the thumb is that the QT interval should be less than half the preceding RR interval. For the sake of simplicity in the range of normal heart rate of 60–100/minute, QT intervals are generally in the range of 0.36–0.44 seconds.

▪ NORMAL PATTERNS AND VARIATIONS OF THE ELECTROCARDIOGRAM

No two individuals have identical electrocardiograms. It is important to know the normal variations and the leads in which they occur.

P wave. P wave is normally upright in lead I, II, V_3 to V_6; upright, biphasic or inverted in V_1 and V_2, and inverted in aVR. Its amplitude should not exceed 2 or *3 mm,* in any lead, and its normal contour is generally rounded. It is generally tallest in lead II.

Q wave. A small Q 1 to 2 mm in amplitude is a usual finding in leads III and aVF and in chest leads over the LV. Deep QS complexes are normal in aVR which shows downward direction of all complexes because the lead faces the cavity of the heart. QS complexes are occasionally found in lead III and leads over the RV. The Q wave normally should not be more than 0.04 second in duration and 3 mm in depth. A deep Q in III may 'be due to a high diaphragm and tends to diminish in size or

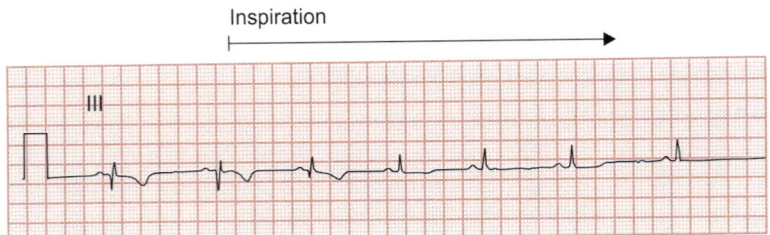

Fig. 8: Electrocardiogram showing disappearance of Q wave with inspiration.

disappear on deep inspiration **(Fig. 8)**. A wide Q_3 not associated with wide or deep Q waves in aVF and II is usually normal. Normally, Q is less than 25% of the succeeding R wave.

QRS Complex. The duration of the normal QRS should not exceed 0.10 sec. If total amplitude above and below the isoelectric line is 5 mm or less in all three standard leads, it is abnormal. Amplitudes up to 20 or 30 mm are occasionally seen in lead II in normal hearts while the generally accepted maximum in precordial lead is 25 or 30 mm.

In lead V_1 the R wave is usually small and the S wave deep, and as one moves across the chest the R wave gradually increases in amplitude and the S wave becomes smaller. Failure of the R wave to increase as the electrode moves across the precordium from right to left is abnormal

S is maximum in amplitude in V_2-V_3 and gradually decreases in size in leads further to the left of the precordium. The intermediate or transition zone is seen at V_3-V_4 where a combination of types of deflections obtained on either side of the precordium is seen.

ST segment. Normally, it is on the same level as the TP segment, i.e., it is isoelectric or only slightly above or below it. It is at times normally elevated not more than 1 mm in standard leads and even 2 mm in some of the chest leads (early repolarisation). Normally, it is not depressed by more than half a millimeter. In shape the ST segment normally curves gently and imperceptibly into the proximal limb of the succeeding T wave. ST segment elevation in the anterior chest leads is a normal variant when it follows an S wave. It is then referred to as 'high take off ST segment.

T wave. Normally upright in I and II and in chest leads over the left ventricle, it is negative or inverted in aVR and often in V_1 and at times in V_2. The T wave is normally upright in aVL and aVF if the QRS is more than 5 mm tall, with smaller R wave in these leads the T wave may be inverted. T waves in V_3-V_6 must be upright. In general in left chest leads, the taller the R wave, taller the T waves should be.

U wave. A small wave of low voltage is sometimes seen following the T wave and is in the same direction as T. It is often best seen in V_2.

■ ELECTROCARDIOGRAPHIC POSITION OF THE HEART

The normal ECG patterns are recorded when the heart is in the normal position. Variations of the positions of the heart in the thoracic cage influence the ECG patterns. The augmented limb leads are especially useful in demonstrating this. The lead aVR however is little influenced by the position of the heart.

Rotation on Anteroposterior Axis (Fig. 9)

Normal or Intermediate Position

Here the left ventricular potentials are transmitted equally to the left shoulder and leg. Hence, the ventricular complexes of both aVL and aVF resemble the left ventricular leads V_5 and V_6.

Horizontal Position

The left ventricle "looks at" the left shoulder and the right ventricle towards the left lower extremity, aVL therefore resembles V_5 and V_6 and aVF resembles V_1 and V_2. This is often seen in pregnancy, obesity and ascites where the diaphragm is elevated.

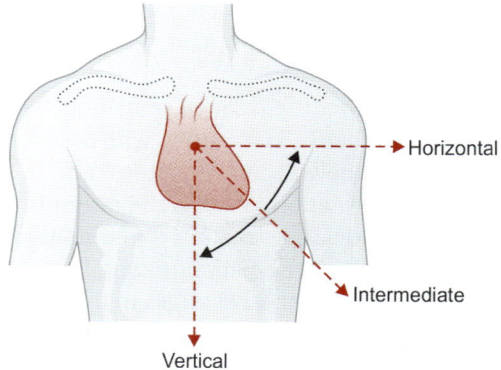

Fig. 9: Rotation of the heart on anteroposterior axis.

14 The Normal Electrocardiogram

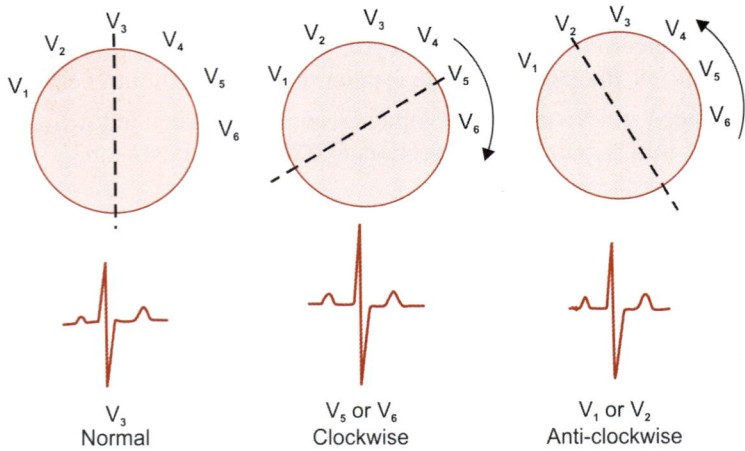

Fig. 10: Rotation of the heart on longitudinal axis.

Vertical Position

Here aVL resembles right precordial leads V_1 and V_2, and a VF resembles left precordial leads V_5 and V_6. This is often seen in thin individuals and in those with an emphysematous chest.

Rotation on Longitudinal Axis (Fig. 10)

Clockwise and Anti-clockwise Rotation

In addition to variations due to rotation on the anteroposterior axis, rotation of the heart may occur on its longitudinal axis **(Fig. 10)**. This rotation is called clockwise when the RV is rotated anteriorly and to the left and anti-clockwise when the LV is rotated anteriorly and to the right. The degree of rotation can be judged from the precordial leads V_1 to V_6.

With *clockwise rotation,* the stage of transition moves further to the left and may appear between V_5 and V_6 with S waves still in V_5, V_6. Extreme clockwise rotation will give rS pattern in V_1 to V_6.

With *anti-clockwise* rotation, there is rS pattern in V_1, V_2, V_3 and qR pattern in V_4 to V_6. Clockwise rotation is frequently present with a vertical heart and anti-clockwise with horizontal heart.

As with vertical and horizontal changes in the electrical axis, the different types of rotation may occur without any organic disease of the heart, although RV enlargement will tend to cause clockwise rotation and LV enlargement anti-clockwise rotation.

CHAPTER 3

Method of Analysis of the Electrocardiogram

Correct recording—Before starting to analyze an ECG, it is necessary to ensure that the record was made correctly by observing the following:
1. **The ECG grid and Standardization:** Horizontal and vertical lines are marked on all ECG papers. The vertical lines represent time and are divided into large and small squares. Every fifth line is marked deeper than the others. Each large square represents 0.2 seconds and each small is one-fifth of this, i.e., 0.04 seconds. The horizontal lines represent voltage, 1 mm being equal to 0.1 millivolt. For correct standardization 1 millivolt of potential difference should give a 10 mm vertical deflection **(Fig. 11)**.
2. **Paper speed:** It should be 25 mm/second. A speed of 50 mm/second will space out the entire PQRST complex.

Interpretation: In the interpretation of an electrocardiogram, it is advisable to follow a method, such as one described below so that the individual features of the tracings are recorded in a definite sequence thus facilitating the diagnosis.

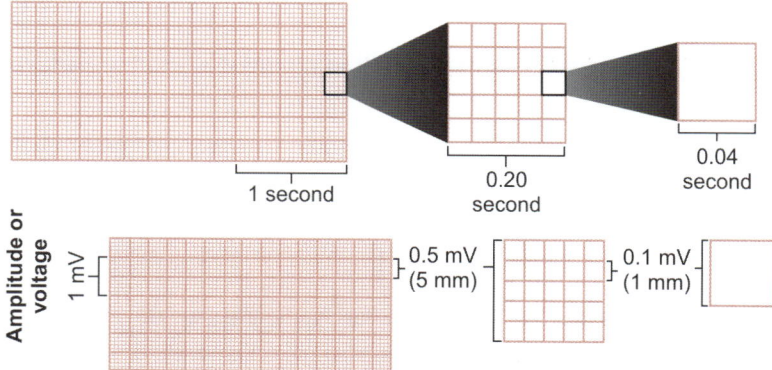

Fig. 11: Time lines, voltage lines and correct standardization in an electrocardiogram.

16 Method of Analysis of the Electrocardiogram

I. Rate
II. Rhythm
III. Voltage
IV. Electrical axis
V. P wave
VI. PR interval
VII. Q wave
VIII. QRS complex
IX. ST segment
X. T wave
XI. QT interval
XII. U wave
XIII. J wave

■ RATE

The rate of the heart per minute can be calculated from the electrocardiogram in the following ways:

Regular rhythm

a. Count the number of 0.2 second time intervals (one big square) between the peaks of any two successive R waves for ventricular rate (or P waves for atrial rate or pacemaker spikes for pacemaker rate). Divide $\frac{60}{0.2}$ = 300 by this figure. In **Figure 12,** there are four 0.2 second time intervals between two successive R waves. Hence, the ventricular rate is about 75 per minute.

b. Count the number of R waves falling in 15 successive big squares (3 seconds) and multiply this by 20, or in 10 big squares and multiply by 30. In **Figure 13,** there are 7 R waves in 15 large squares, therefore, the heart rate per minute is 7 × 20 = 140.

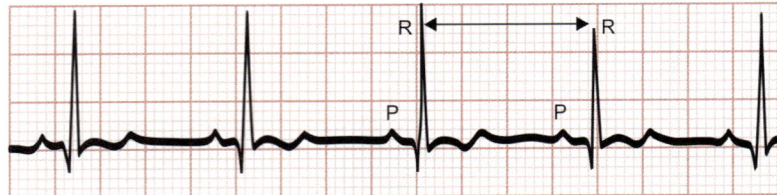

Fig. 12: Measurement of the heart rate, regular rhythm. Determining the time interval between two successive R waves.

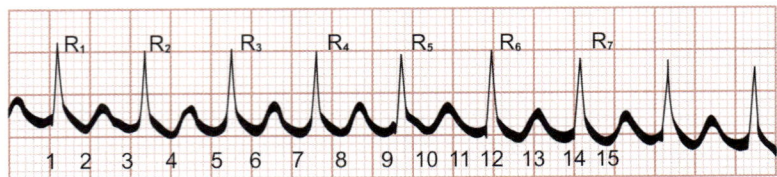

Fig. 13: Measurement of the cardiac rate, regular rhythm. Counting the number of R waves falling in 15 successive 0.2 second intervals.

Method of Analysis of the Electrocardiogram

Number of small squares	Heart rate
5 (1 large square)	300
6	250
7	214
8	188
9	167
10 (2 large squares)	150
11	136
12	125
13	115
14	107
15 (3 large squares)	100
16	94
17	88
18	83
19	79
20 (4 large squares)	75
21	71
22	68
23	65
24	63
25 (5 large squares)	60
26	58
27	56
28	54
29	52
30 (6 large squares)	50
31	48
32	47
33	45
34	44
35 (7 large squares)	43
36	42
37	41
38	39
39	38
40 (8 large squares)	37

   c. Count the number of small squares between 2 R waves and divide 1500 by this number, for heart rate per minute (See above table)

Irregular rhythm (Fig. 14): Count the number of squares over a given period of time, say 3.0 seconds interval. Since, each large square = 0.2

18 Method of Analysis of the Electrocardiogram

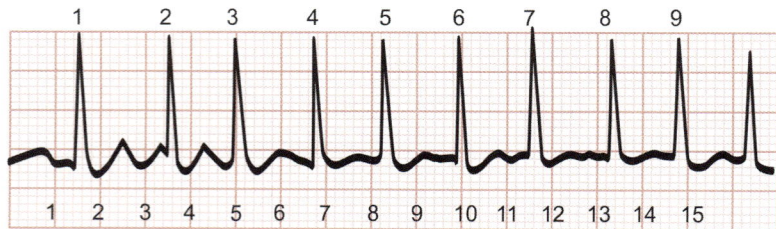

Fig. 14: Determination of heart rate, irregular rhythm. Count the number of complexes (R waves) in span of 15 large squares (3 Secs), in the illustration, the number of R waves is 9, therefore, heart rate/minute = 20 × 9 = 180.

second, 15 large squares = 15 × 0.2 = 3 seconds. Multiply this Figure by 20 to give rate/60 seconds.

■ RHYTHM

For diagnosis of an *arrhythmia,* the following observations must be made:
1. *P waves*—for atrial rhythm.
2. *QRS complexes*—for ventricular rhythm.
3. *Relationship between P waves and QRS complexes*—for atrio-ventricular conduction.
4. *Any unusual complexes*—early, late or of unusual contour.

A. Sinus Rhythm

Sinus rhythm P waves are upright and regular in leads II, III, aVF
1. **Normal sinus rhythm (Fig. 15):** Impulses originate at SA node at normal rate of 60–100/minute.
2. **Sinus bradycardia (Fig. 16):** Heart rate less than 60/minute.
3. **Sinus tachycardia (Fig. 17):** Heart rate more than 100/minute.
   Bradycardia-Tachycardia syndrome (Sick sinus syndrome). The bradycardia-tachy-cardia syndrome, consisting of alternating bradycardia, due to sinus arrest, sinus bradycardia, or sinoatrial exit block combined with tachycardia from paroxysmal atrial or junctional arrhythmias **(Figs. 18A and B)** may produce symptoms referable to the slow or fast heart rates.
4. **Sinus arrhythmia (Fig. 19):** P waves identical and upright in leads II, III, aVF, but rhythmically irregular. Longest PP interval exceeds

Method of Analysis of the Electrocardiogram

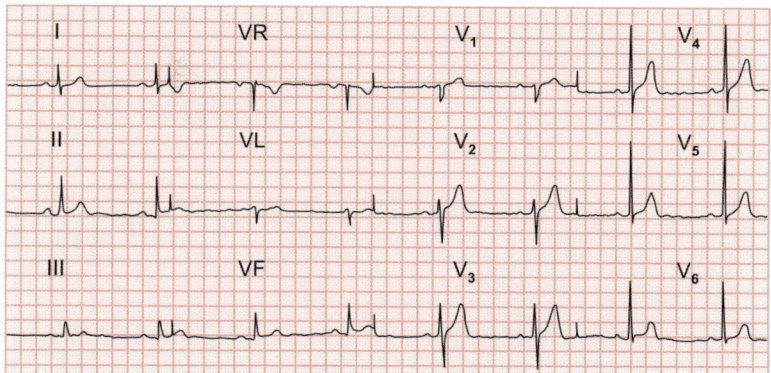

Fig. 15: Normal sinus rhythm.

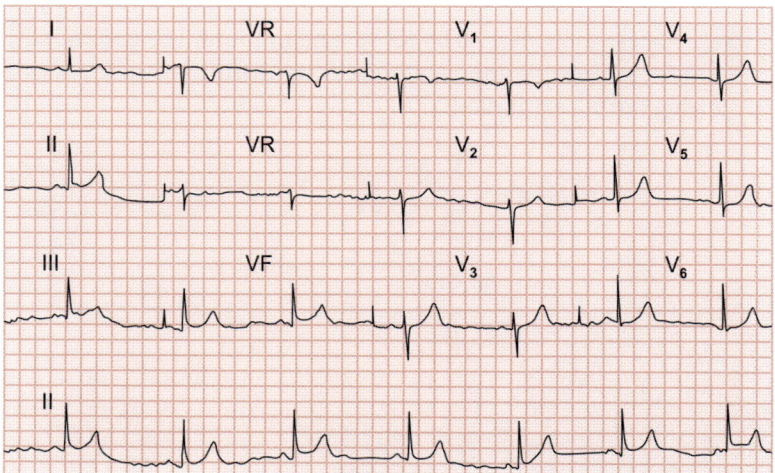

Fig. 16: Sinus bradycardia.

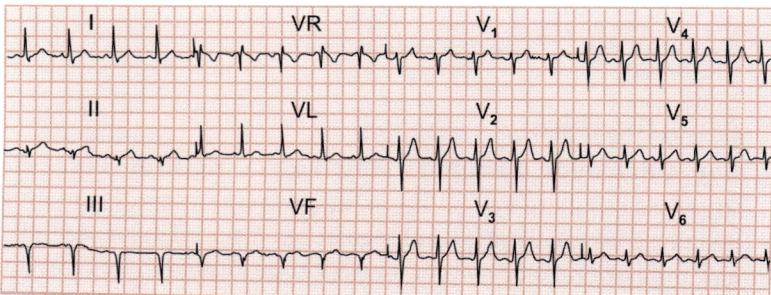

Fig. 17: Sinus tachycardia.

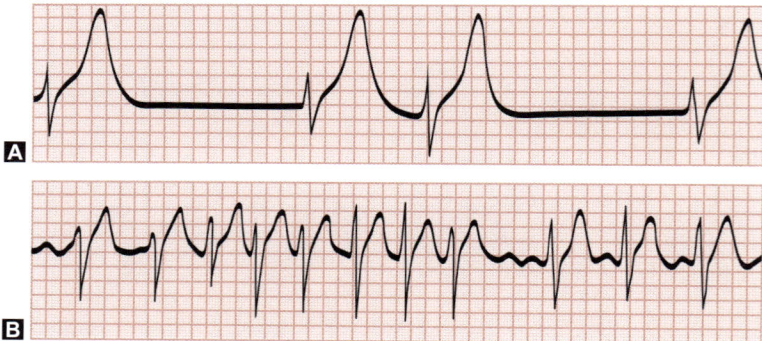

Figs. 18A and B: The 'sick sinus syndrome': (A) Irregular nodal bradycardia; (B) Paroxysmal atrial tachycardia.

the shortest such interval by 0.1 second or more. The commonest form is *respiratory*, the rate increasing during inspiration and slowing during expiration.

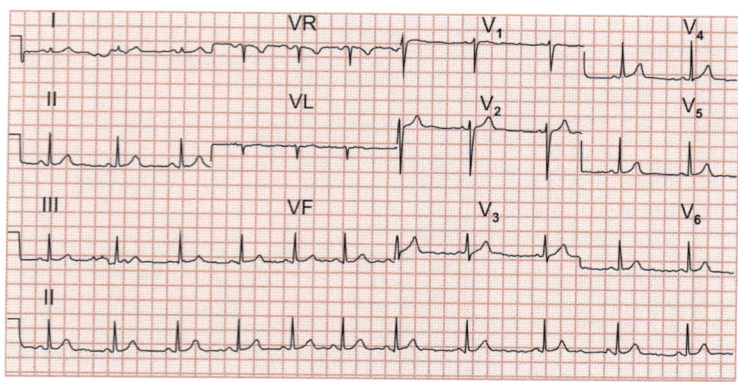

Fig. 19: Sinus arrhythmia. The first part of the tracing is during expiration and inspiration increases the rate.

B. Atrial Rhythms

1. **Non-sinus node (coronary sinus) atrial rhythm (Fig. 20):** Impulses originate low in the atrium, travel retrograde and also distally. P waves identical and regular but inverted in leads, II, III, aVF implying an origin other than SA node located in upper right corner of the atrium.

Method of Analysis of the Electrocardiogram

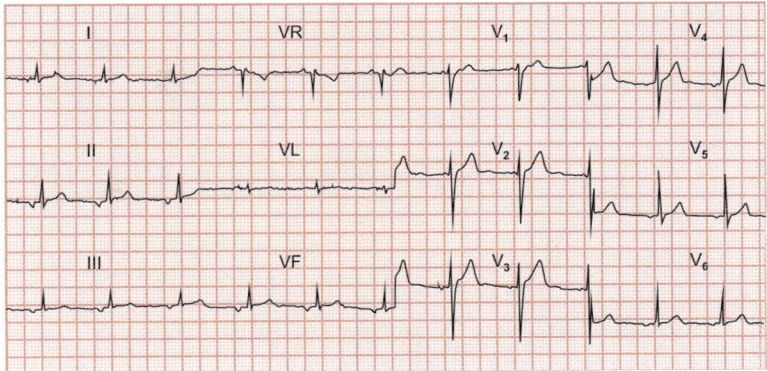

Fig. 20: Non-sinus node atrial rhythm.

2. **Wandering atrial pacemaker (Fig. 21)**: Impulses originate from various foci in atria. The shape or contour of P wave varies from beat to beat in a single lead, often associated with variation of PR interval and PP (and RR) intervals.

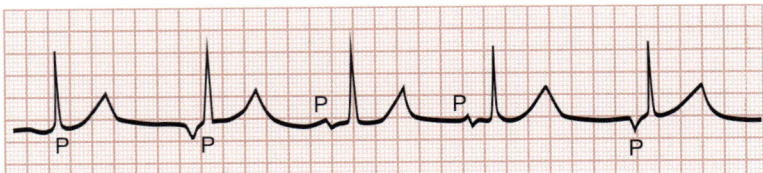

Fig. 21: Wandering atrial pacemaker, variation in P wave contour, PR interval, PP and hence RR intervals.

3. **Multifocal atrial tachycardia (Fig. 22)**: Impulses originate rapidly and irregularly at different points in atria. MAT is similar to wandering pacemaker, but the difference is that the heart rate is usually more than 100/minute. It is usually associated with severe pulmonary disease often with respiratory decompensation or congestive heart failure (CHF).
4. **Paroxysmal atrial tachycardia (Figs. 23A and B):** Impulses recycle repeatedly in and in vicinity of AV node due to slowing in area of unidirectional block (re-entry tachycardia). P waves regular, identical in lead II, sometimes merged with T waves and very rapid rate (usually 160–220/minute).

If the rate is sufficiently rapid in PAT, normal refractoriness of the A-V junction may prevent transmission of many stimuli—atrial

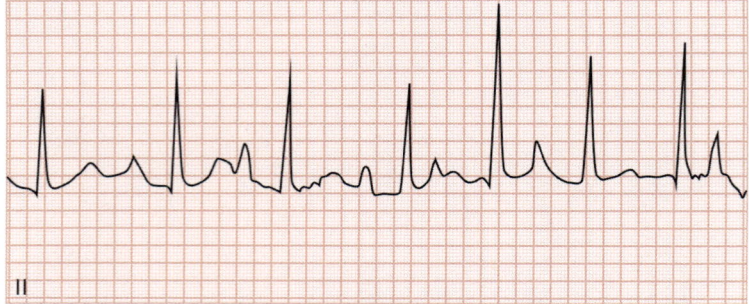

Fig. 22: Multifocal atrial tachycardia. P wave contours, PR, PP and thus RR intervals may all vary.

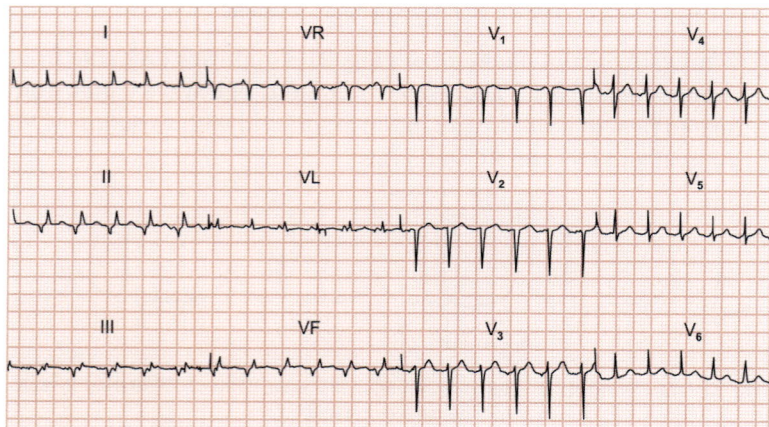

Fig. 23A: Paroxysmal atrial tachycardia (PAT). P waves regular and inverted.

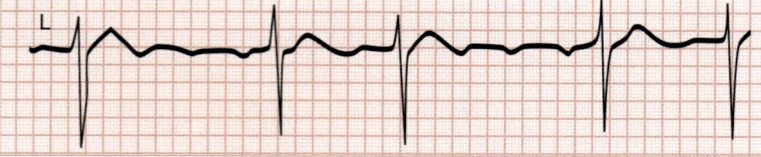

Fig. 23B: Paroxysmal atrial tachycardia with varying AV block. Note the irregular ventricular rate.

tachycardia with varying block **(Fig. 23B)**. This arrhythmia is often due to digitalis toxicity.

5. **Atrial fibrillation (Figs. 24A and B):** Impulses follow chaotic, random pathway in atria. P waves not seen because of lack of

effective pumping motion of the atria. QRS complexes irregularly irregular. The base line may be coarsely or finely irregular. The ventricular rate may be rapid or slow.

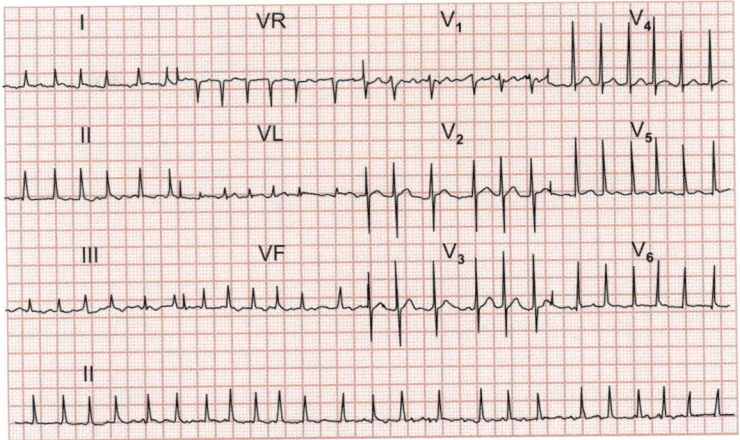

Fig. 24A: Atrial fibrillation with rapid rate.

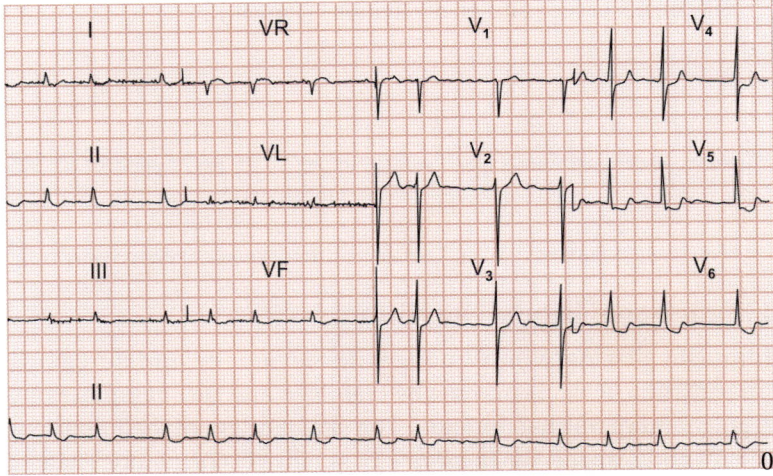

Fig. 24B: Slow atrial fibrillation. Digitalis effect.

6. **Atrial flutter (Fig. 25):** Impulses travel in a circular course in the atria, setting up regular, rapid (220–300/minute) flutter waves. Rapid, identical undulating P waves of longer duration and at times

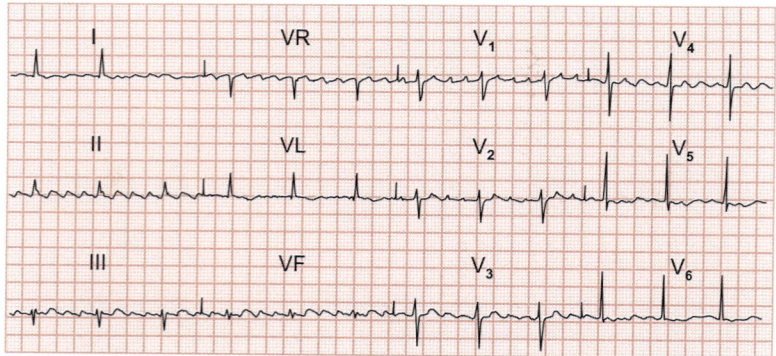

Fig. 25: Atrial flutter with 4:1 block. The rhythm is regular rate is slow, QRS duration normal.

of longer amplitudes than normal P waves (flutter or F waves). The F waves have a rate of about 300/minute, but depending on the AV block which is usually present, the rate may be 150 (2:1 block), 100 (3:1 block), or 75 (4:1 block) per minute. The baseline of atrial flutter is never isoelectric. Coarse atrial fibrillation may at times resemble atrial flutter and a rhythm with characteristics of both may be observed (Flutter-fibrillation) **(Fig. 26)**.

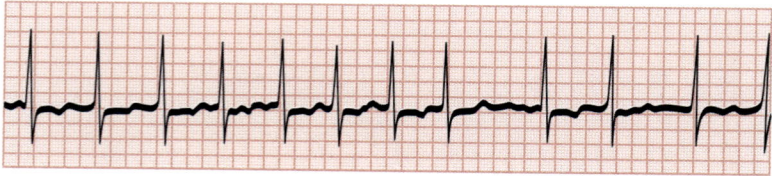

Fig. 26: Atrial flutter-fibrillation. Combination of flutter and fibrillation waves.

C. Junctional (Nodal) Rhythm

Impulses originate in AV node with retrograde and antegrade transmission. P waves may not be identified and QRS complexes are regular and of normal duration. The site of origin of the impulse is the AV node, hence, the heart rate is usually 40–60/minute. (Rate of junctional cells is lower than the rate of SA node). P waves in leads II, III, aVF tend to be inverted (because impulses that originate in AV node are transmitted in a retrograde direction to the atrium). Depending on whether the junctional rhythm reaches and depolarizes the atrium before, at the same time or after the ventricles, the P wave will precede, be buried in or follow QRS complex **(Fig. 27)**.

Method of Analysis of the Electrocardiogram — 25

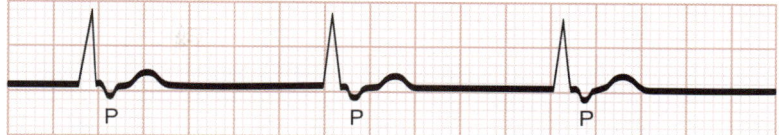

Fig. 27: Junctional rhythm. P waves inverted and follow QRS. Rate slow. QRS duration normal.

D. Ventricular Rhythms

a. **Idioventricular rhythm (Fig. 28):** The rhythm originates from the ventricle itself. QRS complexes are wide, often somewhat bizarre with T waves in opposite direction to QRS complexes and with rate of 20–40/minute.

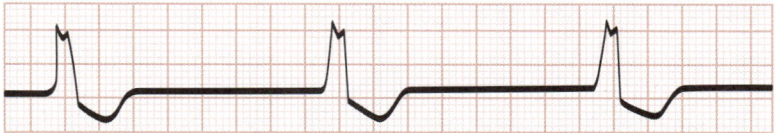

Fig. 28: Idioventricular rhythm. Total absence of P wave. RR interval regular.

Accelerated idioventricular rhythm (Slow ventricular tachycardia)—Wide, often bizarre **QRS** complexes with rate usually between 80-120/minute **(Fig. 29).**

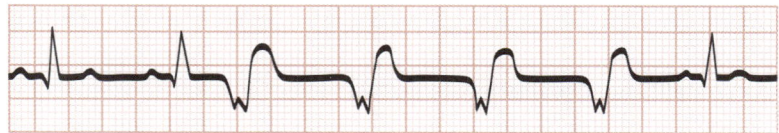

Fig. 29: Accelerated idioventricular rhythm (AIVR).

b. **Ventricular tachycardia (Fig. 30):** Rapid, broad and often bizarre QRS complexes with rates above 140/minute.
c. **Torsade de pointes ventricular tachycardia (Fig. 31):** It is an uncommon arrhythmia characterised by a ventricular tachycardia, often of moderate rate but associated with an undulating QRS height due to a slow but continual variation in the QRS axis (polymorphic **VT**). Its importance is due to its precipitation by antiarrhythmic drugs, particularly if electrolyte disturbances coexist, along with prolonged QT interval.

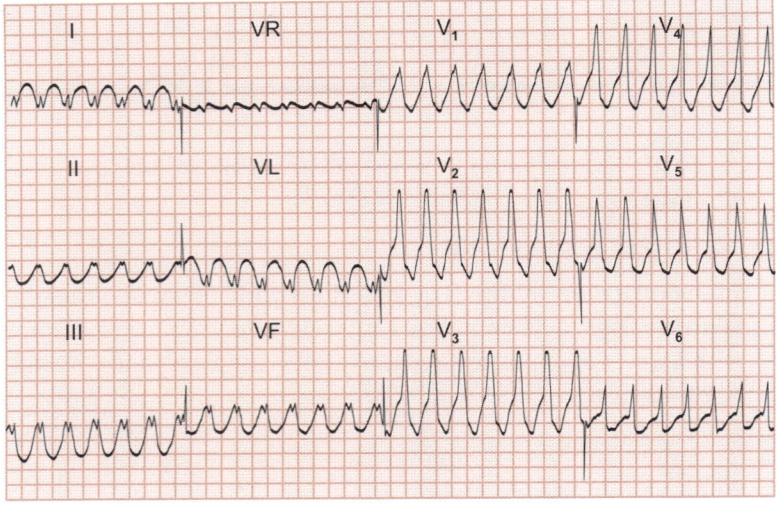

Fig. 30: Ventricular Tachycardia (VT).

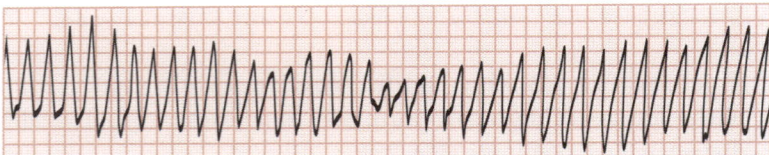

Fig. 31: Drug-induced ventricular tachycardia of the torsade de pointes type. Note the variation in the axis of the QRS complex causing an undulated (or twisted) appearance.

d. **Ventricular fibrillation (Fig. 32):** There is chaotic ventricular depolarization. There are no true QRS complexes and the ECG baseline shows coarse or fine chaotic undulations.

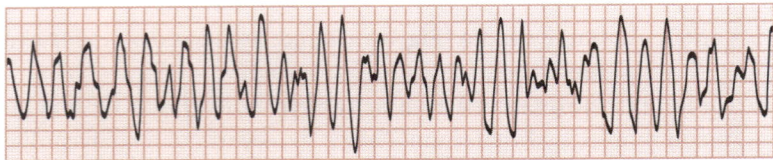

Fig. 32: Ventricular fibrillation. Complete absence of properly formed ventricular complexes.

e. **Pacemaker rhythm (Fig. 33):** Transvenous pacemaker produces a beat in the right ventricle; and therefore a wide QRS. Besides wide QRS complexes, the pacemaker discharge itself produces a pacemaker 'spike', seen as a narrow vertical line at the onset of the QRS complex.

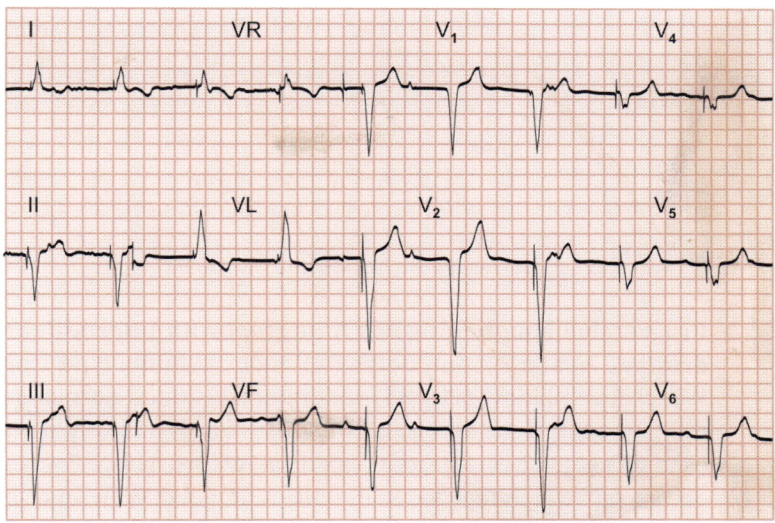

Fig. 33: Pacemaker rhythm. Note the pacemaker spike.

E. Atrioventricular Conduction Variations

AV conduction is assessed by examining the relationship between P waves and QRS complexes. The basic thing to observe is whether P waves are always related to QRS complexes, sometimes related to QRS complexes or never related to QRS complexes.

1. **Fixed normal PR interval:** P waves precede QRS complexes by normal fixed PR interval—normal sinus rhythm **(Fig. 15)**.
2. **Fixed but short PR interval:**
   a. Junctional or coronary sinus rhythm **(Fig. 20)**.
   b. Wolff-Parkinson-White syndrome **(Fig. 64)**.
   c. Lown Ganong Levine syndrome **(Fig. 62)**.
3. **P wave related to each QRS complex but variable PR interval:**
   a. Wandering atrial pacemaker **(Fig. 21)**.
   b. Multifocal atrial tachycardia **(Fig. 22)**.
4. **Fixed but prolonged (>0.2 sec) PR interval**: First degree AV block **(Fig. 34)**.

28 Method of Analysis of the Electrocardiogram

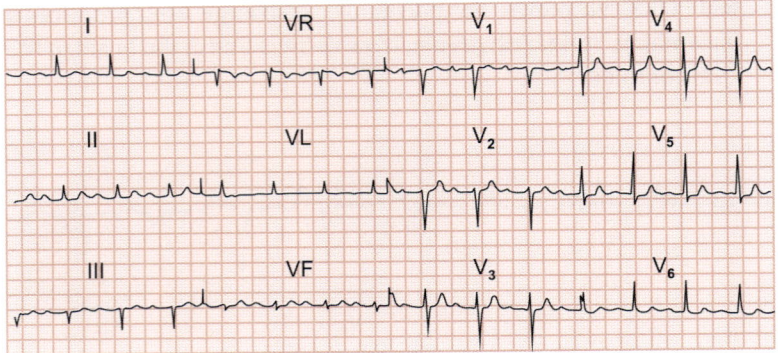

Fig. 34: First degree heart block. PR interval 0.28 sec.

5. a. **Progressive lengthening of PR interval with intermittent dropped beats:** Second degree AV block (Mobitz type 1 or Wenckebach block) **(Fig. 35)**—PR interval is often normal in the first beat of the series, but lengthens progressively with each successive beat until conduction at AV node fails, a P wave occurs, fails to conduct and so the QRS is dropped. With a pause between QRS complexes, AV nodal conduction recovers and the next PR interval is normal again.

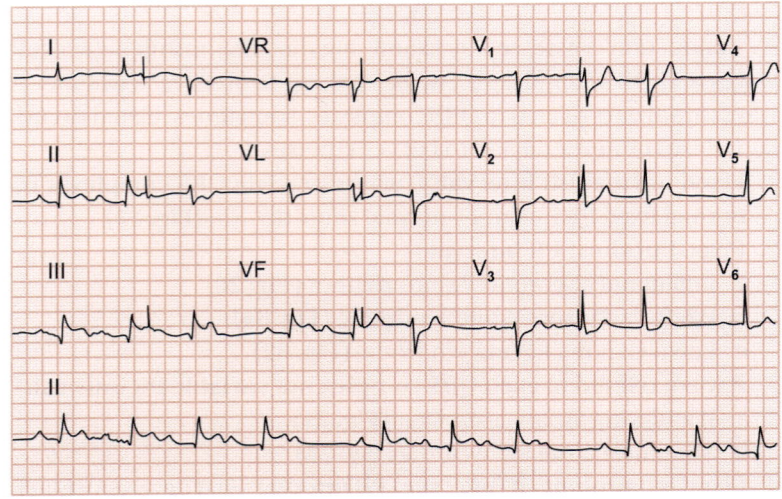

Fig. 35: Progressive lengthening of PR interval followed by "dropped QRS". Mobitz type 1 (Wenckebach).

b. **PR intervals are constant and then a P wave suddenly fails to conduct:** Second degree AV block (Mobitz type 2) **(Fig. 36)**. Here the AV block is lower (at level of bundle of His, bundle branches, or at the level of the fascicles).

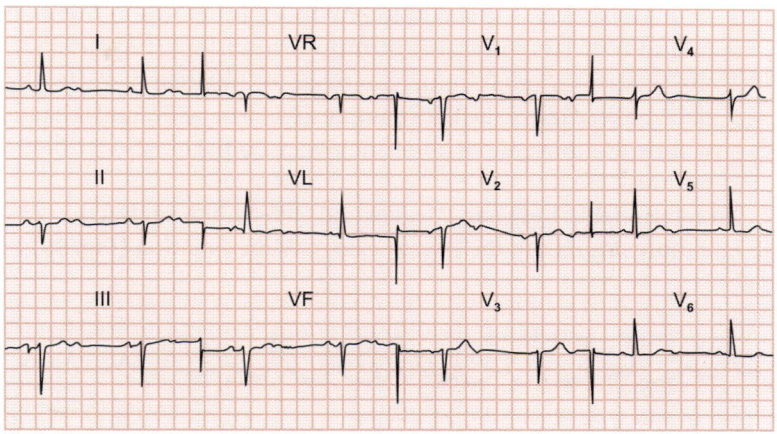

Fig. 36: Mobitz type 2 AV block. (Non- Wenckebach).

c. **PR interval remains constant,** but the ventricles respond to every second **(Fig. 37)**, third or fourth beat—2:1, 3:1, 4:1, block. When the conduction is 3:1 or 4:1 the block is termed high grade AV block. Pulse slow and regular.

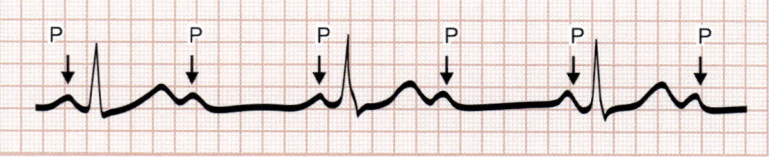

Fig. 37: 2:1 AV block.

6. **No relationship between P waves and QRS complexes,** which are regular, but at a slower rate than the P waves—third-degree (complete) AV block **(Fig. 38)**.

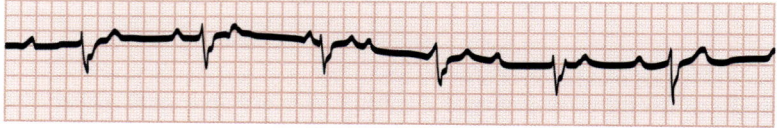

Fig. 38: Complete heart block.

a. *High AV block:* If complete AV block occurs above AV node, a junctional rhythm will take over and drive the ventricles, producing narrow QRS complexes at the intrinsic rate of AV node, usually about 40–55/minute.
b. *Low AV block:* If the site of the AV block is below the AV node (bundle of His, bilateral bundle branch or trifascicular), the ventricles must be driven from an intrinsic ventricular pacemaker. Hence the QRS complexes will be wide, and the rate will be the intrinsic of a ventricular pacemaker, about 20-40/minute.

7. **No relationship between P waves** and QRS complexes but the QRS rate more rapid than the P wave rate—AV dissociation **(Fig. 39)**.

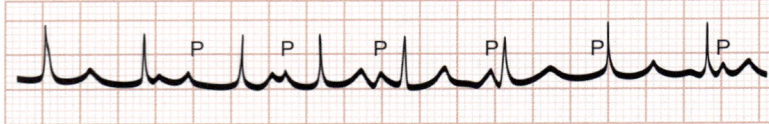

Fig. 39: AV disssociation. The ventricles beat independently at a slightly faster rate than the atria and the PR interval gets shorter and shorter. The last P wave can be seen to have 'walked through' QRS.

F. Unusual Complexes or Beats

Complexes may be unusual in terms of either contour or timing. If the shape of a QRS complex differs in the same lead, it should be determined whether the unusual complex is of atrial, junctional or ventricular origin.

a. **Premature contraction occurs early** before next sinus beat is expected in a regular rhythm:
  1. *Atrial* **(Fig. 40)**: P wave contour is slightly different from other sinus beats. QRS complexes are normal except for timing.

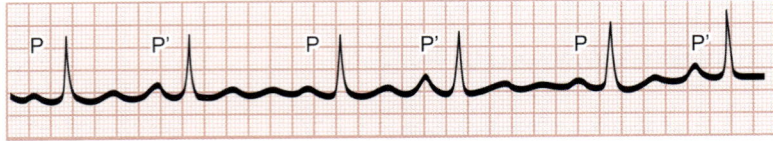

Fig. 40: Tracing showing atrial premature beat (P') after each normal beat (P)—atrial bigeminy. Note the alteration in the shape of the P waves of the premature contractions. The compensatory pause is incomplete.

2. *Junctional (Nodal)* **(Fig. 41)**: As in case of junctional rhythm, the P wave may precede (usually with a short PR interval), be buried in, or follow the QRS which is narrow with contour similar to that of other QRS complexes in all leads.

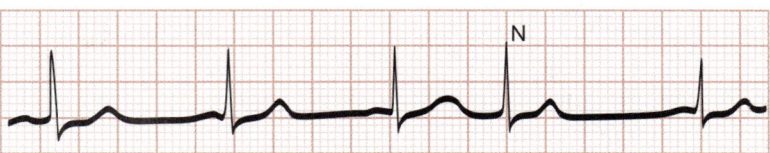

Fig. 41: Junctional (Nodal) premature contraction (N). There is no P wave before the premature beat and the QRS complex resembles the others. The compensatory pause is complete.

3. *Ventricular* **(Figs. 42A to C)**: QRS wider than normal and distorted in shape. There is usually no P wave. The T wave following the premature beat is in the opposite direction to the main deflection of the QRS complex. Sum of the RR intervals immediately before and after the ventricular premature beat is equal to the sum of two regular RR intervals, i.e., the premature contraction is completely compensatory.

Premature beats arising from different parts of the ventricles show different forms **(Fig. 43)**: Multifocal ventricular premature beats.

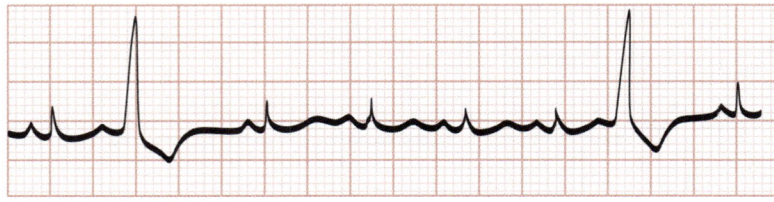

Fig. 42A: Ventricular premature beats with full compensatory pauses. Note the R on T phenomenon.

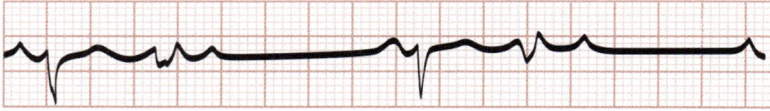

Fig. 42B: Electrocardiogram showing ventricular premature beats causing coupling or bigeminy.

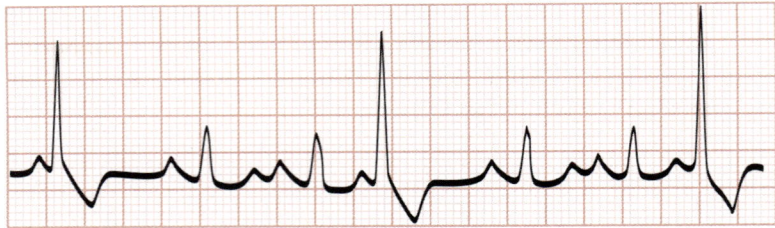

Fig. 42C:. Trigeminy. After every two normal beats, there is a ventricular premature beat.

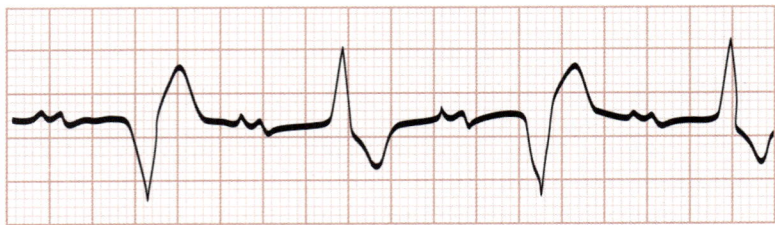

Fig. 43: Ventricular premature beats arising alternately from two different foci.

4. *Interpolated premature beat:* The premature beat occurs so early in diastole that the next normal atrial impulse finds the conduction tissues and ventricles ready to respond. The premature beat occurs midway between two normal sinus beats without any compensatory pause—interpolated ventricular premature beat **(Fig. 44)**.

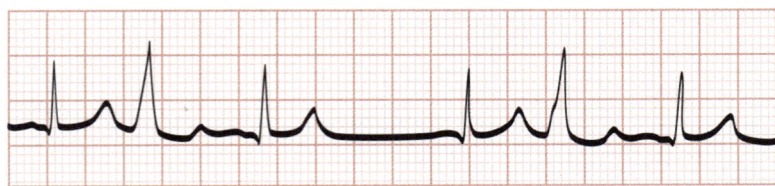

Fig. 44: Interpolated premature beats. The ventricular premature beat is interposed between two normal beats without compensatory pause.

b. **Sinus pause and sinus arrest:** The SA node itself may pause and the rhythm may resume with another sinus beat. If the interval between sinus beats is short (1–2 seconds) or less it is labeled as *sinus pause.* If it is a longer pause, it is called *sinus arrest* (SA block) **(Fig. 45)**.

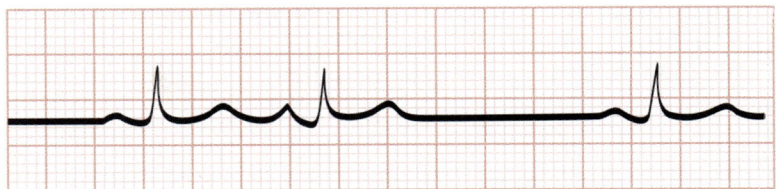

Fig. 45: SA block. A complete PQRST complex is omitted and the PP interval is twice the normal length.

When the SA node fails to initiate an impulse one of the following may occur:
1. *SA node resumes:* The SA node again takes over and a normal rhythm is restored **(Fig. 46)**. Here the resulting pause is not an exact multiple of the cycle length.

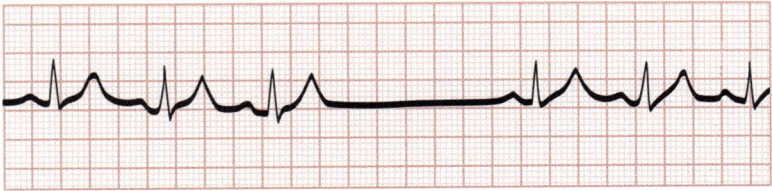

Fig. 46: Sinus arrest. The SA node again takes over and normal rhythm is restored,

2. *Escape beats:*
   a. Atrial escape beat **(Fig. 47)**: An ectopic focus in the atria may fire an impulse after such a pause, stimulating the atria. Conduction then proceeds down through the AV node normally.

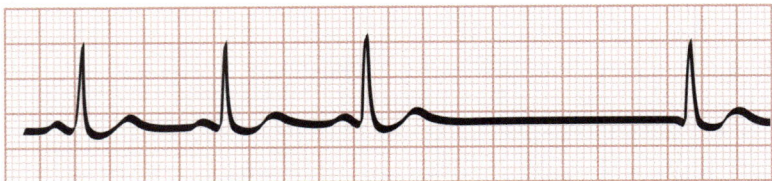

Fig. 47: Atrial escape beat.

   b. Junctional (nodal) escape beat **(Fig. 48)**: Failure of SA node to initiate the cardiac impulse may result in take over by the AV node, usually after 1.2–1.6 seconds.

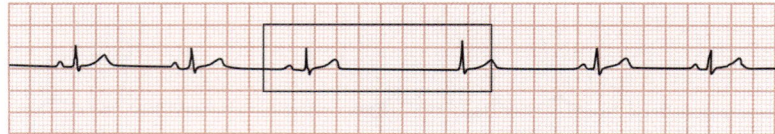

Fig. 48: Sinus arrest with junctional (nodal) escape beat not preceded by a P wave and resembling normal ventricular complex preceded by prolonged period of absent sinus activity.

   c. Ventricular escape beat **(Fig. 49)**: If the SA node and AV node fail, automatic cells in the ventricle must take over (usually after 1.8–2.2 seconds) or 'escape' from their usual control by higher pacemaker in order to maintain the heart beat. Wide, slow QRS complexes with a contour different from that of a normal sinus beat is observed.

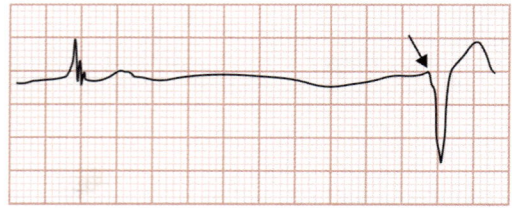

Fig. 49: Sinus arrest with ventricular escape. An abnormal QRS without a preceding P wave.

3. *Idioventricular rhythm:* If the ventricular escape continues for two or more beats, it is designated idioventricular rhythm **(Fig. 28).** It is usually a relatively slow regular rhythm. The QRS complex is widened as the site of impulse formation is usually below the bundle of His.
4. *Ventricular standstill may continue resulting* in death.

■ VOLTAGE

As a rule the term refers to the voltage of the R wave. Normally, the amplitude of the R wave in lead I is less than 16 mm, in aVL 11 mm or less, in aVF 20 mm or less, and in V_5, V_6 less than 26 mm.

High voltage: Causes—
1. Left ventricular hypertrophy
2. Thin chest wall especially in children
3. Bundle branch block sometimes
4. Wolff-Parkinson-White (WPW) syndrome

Low voltage: Low voltage is said to be present when the largest QRS deflection in standard and unipolar limb leads is less than 5 mm, and less than 8 mm in precordial leads. Causes of low voltage are —
1. Old age and cachexia
2. Obesity, thick chest wall or emphysema
3. Pericardial effusion **(Fig. 50)** or constrictive pericarditis
4. Myxedema
5. Diffuse ischemic heart disease
6. Cardiac failure
7. Cardiomyopathy
8. Generalized edema
9. Incorrect standardization

Changing voltage: It is seen in a condition labeled "ELECTRICAL ALTERNANS" in which alternate QRS complexes (and occasionally T waves) are large and small **(Fig. 51)**. Electrical alternans has the same prognostic significance as pulsus alternans.

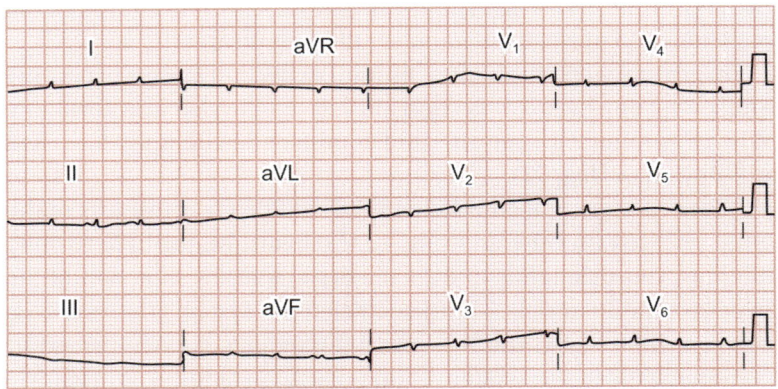

Fig. 50: ECG in pericardial effusion. Note the generalized low voltage.

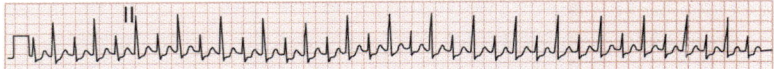

Fig. 51: Electrical alternans.

■ ELECTRICAL AXIS

Depolarization of the ventricles, it was shown earlier can be represented by a small initial force from left to right, followed by a

36 Method of Analysis of the Electrocardiogram

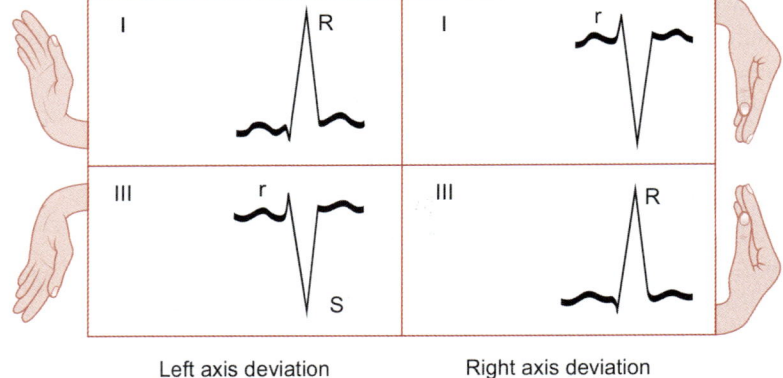

Left axis deviation   Right axis deviation

Fig. 52: Left and right axis deviation as determined by the standard leads I and III.

large force or forces from right to left. The average or mean direction of these forces can be represented by a single force—the mean frontal plane QRS electrical axis. The electrical axis represents the direction of conduction of electrical impulses through the heart.

In general when the highest upward deflection R wave occurs in I and lowest downward deflection in III, it signifies left axis deviation. When a dominant S is seen in I and dominant R in III, it signifies right axis deviation **(Fig. 52)**.

There is a general correlation between the electrical axis of the QRS complex and the anatomy of the heart. Major hypertrophy of either ventricle tends to displace the axis in the direction of the hypertrophied ventricle. The triaxial reference system is formed from unipolar limb leads, and the hexaxial reference system formed by combining the triaxial system of unipolar and standard limb leads.

Procedure for Determining the Electrical Axis

1. **Triaxial reference (vectorial) system:** The axis can be more precisely determined from any two limb leads. By taking the three sides of the standard limb leads and arranging them so that they intersect each other, a triaxial reference system is obtained. The axis on the line corresponding to lead I pointing to the right = 0° and that pointing to left = 180°. All axes above this line are negative and those below are positive. The electrical axis may be determined to

Method of Analysis of the Electrocardiogram

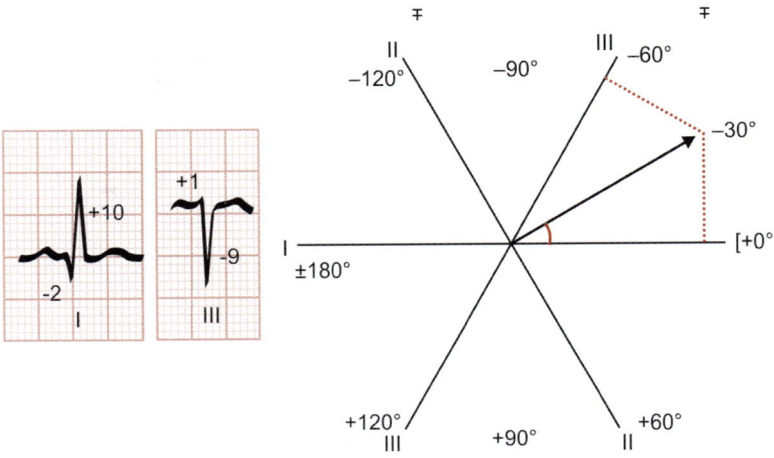

Fig. 53: Measurement of axis deviation, by triaxial reference system.

the nearest 30° by using leads I and III. For example, in **Figure 53**. The net algebraic sum of lead I is –2 +10 = +8, and of lead III +1 –9 = –8. These are plotted along the axis of each lead. Perpendiculars are drawn from these plotted points. A line is then, drawn from the center of the triaxial system to the point of intersection of the two perpendiculars. This represents the mean QRS axis or vector. It is seen that the angle (direction) is –30°.

2. **Hexaxial reference system**: Adding the unipolar leads to the triaxial system reduces the angular separation of the leads to 30° **(Fig. 54)**. The triaxial method, although precise, is cumbersome for routine use. An approximate method can be used to quickly determine the axis by inspection. The method depends on the fact that a positive QRS complex in any given lead means the axis is directed towards the positive pole of that lead, while a negative QRS complex means the axis is directed away from the positive pole of that lead. The relationship of unipolar to bipolar leads is as follows—aVF is the perpendicular of lead I, aVL of lead II, and aVR that of lead III.

In determining the mean electrical axis, it is useful to study the leads I and aVF in order to determine the quadrant in which the vector will be situated **(Fig. 54)**.

Method of Analysis of the Electrocardiogram

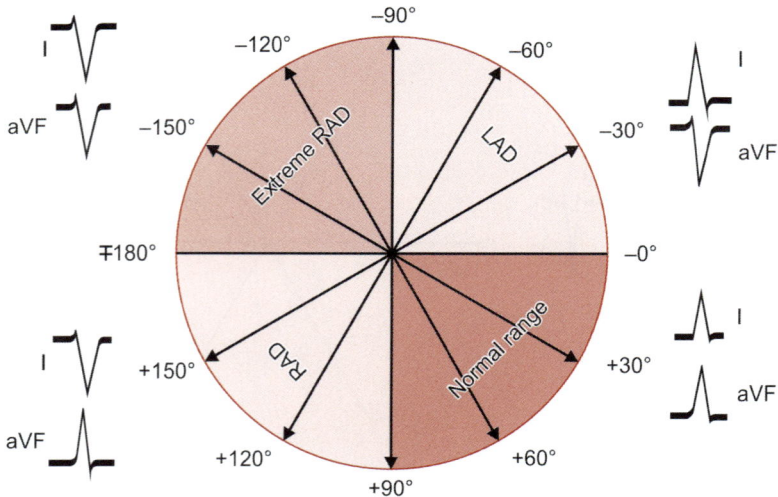

Fig. 54: The hexaxial reference system and range of axis. Determining the mean axis by looking at the QRS complex in I and aVF.

I	aVF	Quadrant
Upright	Upright	0° to 90°
Upright	Inverted	–00 to –90°
Inverted	Upright	90° to 180°
Inverted	Inverted	–90° to –180°

Axis deviation: The axis lies at right angles to the lead with minimal or biphasic deflection and between the two leads with a maximal R deflection.

Normal range: 0° to + 110° in age <40 years. -30 to + 90° in age >40 years.

Left axis deviation	Right axis deviation
1. Physiological—horizontal heart position, pregnancy, stocky build or obesity, abdominal distension	1. Physiological—clockwise rotation of heart, infants up to 6 months of age
2. Hypertrophy and dilatation of LV	2. Hypertrophy and dilatation of RV
3. Inferior wall myocardial infarction	3. Anterolateral cardiac infarction
4. Left bundle branch block	4. Right bundle branch block
5. WPW syndrome type B	5. WPW syndrome type A

Left axis deviation	Right axis deviation
6. Left anterior hemiblock	6. Left posterior hemiblock
7. Tricuspid atresia	7. Dextrocardia
8. Right apical pacing	8. Mediastinal shift to left

Axis indeterminate: (either extreme left or extreme right): between 180° and –120°. S waves seen in all three standard leads (S_1, S_2, S_3 syndrome). Causes—(1) Normal variation occasionally; (2) Cor pulmonale; (3) Some varieties of congenital heart disease.

■ P WAVE ABNORMALITIES

A. Duration and Amplitude: Chamber Enlargement

P mitrale (left atrial enlargement): The normal P wave has two components—the first or right atrial component and the second left atrial component. Normally, these two overlap closely resulting in a pyramid-shaped P wave **(Fig. 55)**. In LA enlargement, the second or left atrial component is delayed resulting in a wide and notched P wave in lead II. In lead V_1 the P wave is biphasic with prominent negative component or mainly negative **(Fig. 56A)** since the left atrium lies behind the right.

P pulmonale (Right atrial enlargement): The right atrial component is increased resulting in tall peaked P wave **(Fig. 56B)**. The P is referred to as P pulmonale or congenitale since it is associated with RA strain in pulmonary hypertension or cyanotic congenital heart disease. In V_1, and V_2, there are tall peaked P waves, as the right atrial force is

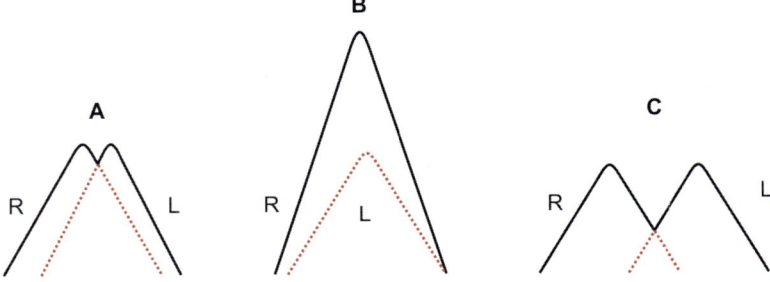

Fig. 55: Diagram to show the components of the P wave. The initial portion of the P wave is produced primarily by the right atrium (R) and the terminal portion by the left atrium (L).—A. B—P pulmonale. C—P mitrale.

40 Method of Analysis of the Electrocardiogram

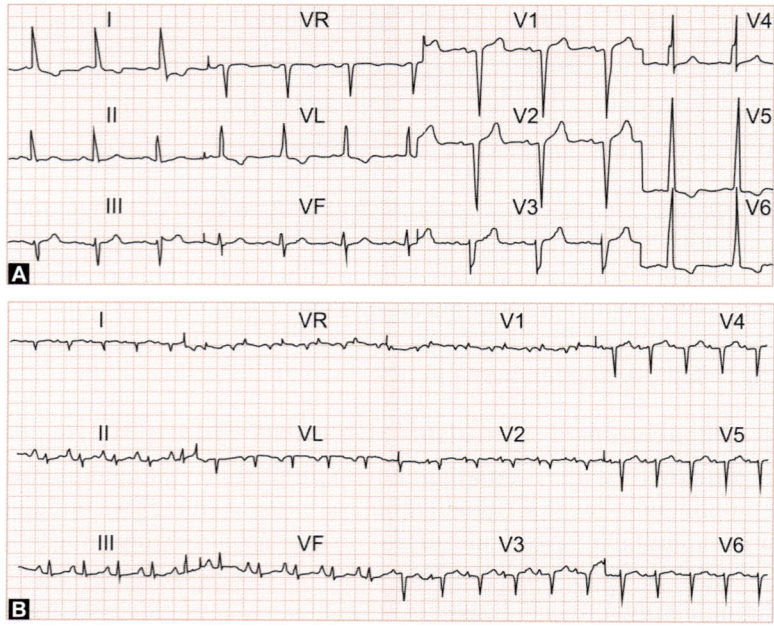

Figs. 56A and B: (A) Left atrial enlargemant. Broad, bifid P in II, mainly negative P in V1 – P mitrale; (B) Right atrial enlargement. Tall and peaked P in II and V1 – P pulmonale.

directed towards these leads. These changes are best seen in lead II since both atrial forces run parallel to the lead.

Biatrial P waves (Biatrial enlargement): When both left and right atria are hypertrophied, there is increase in both amplitude and duration of P wave. In lead II, P is tall and broad, and in V_1, the positive deflection is taller and negative deflection broader **(Fig. 57)**.

B. Absent (Unidentifiable) P waves

1. Atrial fibrillation—replaced by fibrillary waves **(Fig. 58)**
2. Atrial flutter—replaced by flutter or 'F' waves **(Fig. 25)**
3. Sinus arrest **(Fig. 45)**
4. Junctional (AV nodal) rhythm **(Fig. 27)** (P waves may be hidden within QRS complexes).
5. P partially or wholly buried in QRS and T:
    i. Supraventricular paroxysmal tachycardia **(Fig. 59)**
    ii. Supraventricular premature beats **(Fig. 40)**
6. Hyperkalemia **(Fig. 60)**

Method of Analysis of the Electrocardiogram

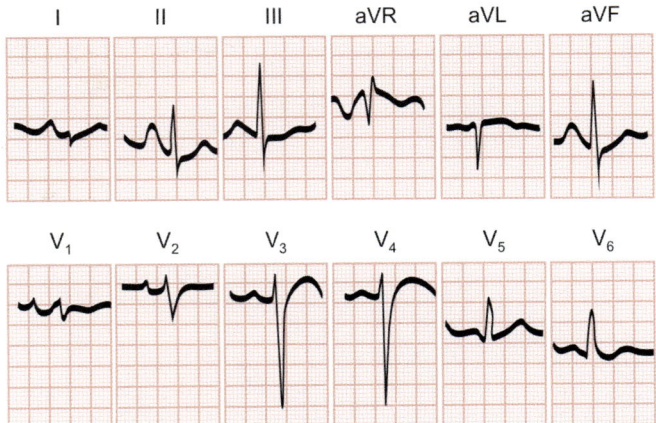

Fig. 57: Biatrial P waves in combined atrial enlargement. The P waves are abnormally broad and tall.

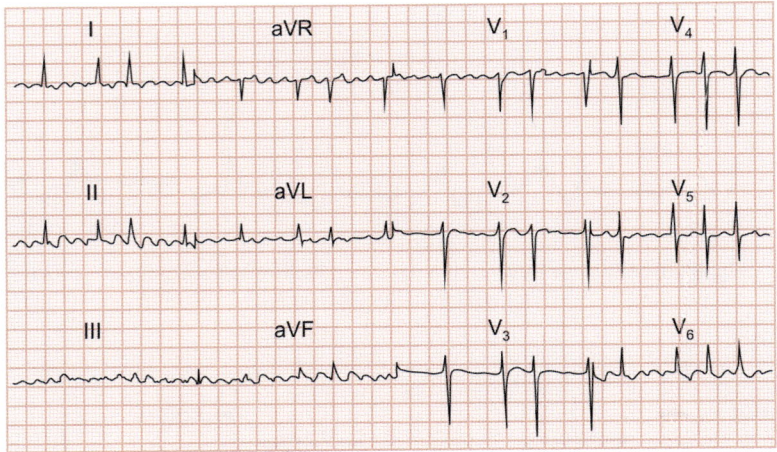

Fig. 58: Atrial fibrillary waves.

C. Inverted P Waves

1. Mirror image dextrocardia—P inverted in lead I along with the QRST complex **(Fig. 61)**, and upright in aVR
2. Atrial premature beats **(Fig. 40)**
3. Atrial tachycardia
4. Junctional rhythm **(Fig. 27)**
5. Non-sinus (Coronary sinus) rhythm **(Fig. 20)**

Method of Analysis of the Electrocardiogram

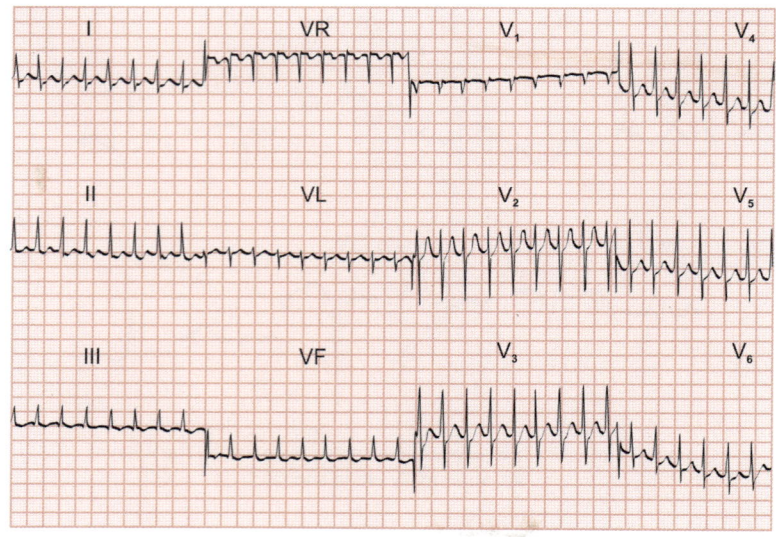

Fig. 59: P waves probably buried in QRS or T in supraventricular paroxysmal tachycardia.

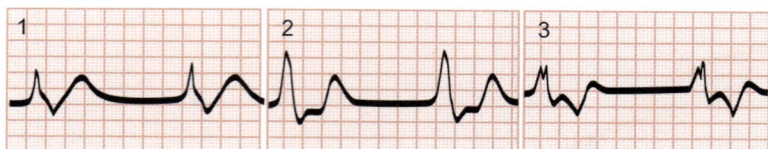

Fig. 60: Hyperkalemia (advanced). Note absent P waves, tall peaked T waves, and widened QRS complexes.

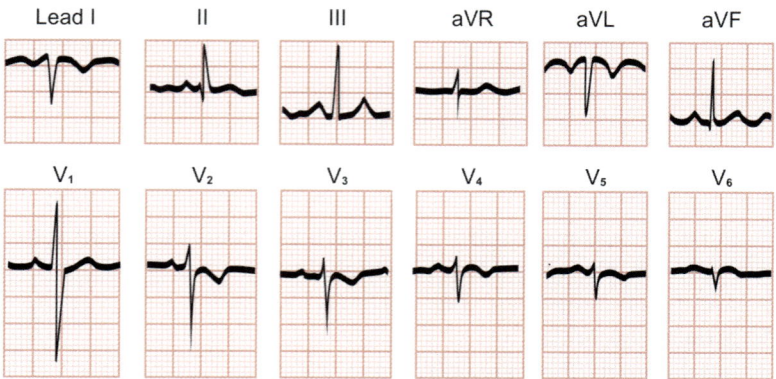

Fig. 61: Dextrocardia. Lead I shows inverted P wave and inverted QRS complex and T wave. This pattern is the mirror image of the usual one found in normal lead I.

D. Changing Shape
Wandering pacemaker **(Fig. 21)**
Atrial ectopics **(Fig. 40)**

■ PR INTERVAL ABNORMALITIES

A. Prolonged
1. First degree heart, block **(Fig. 34)**
2. Hyperkalemia

B. Shortened
1. Junctional rhythm (if P wave precedes the QRS)
2. Short PR interval with wide QRS—WPW syndrome **(Fig. 64)**
3. Short PR interval and normal QRS interval without delta wave—Lown-Ganong-Levine syndrome **(Fig. 62)**

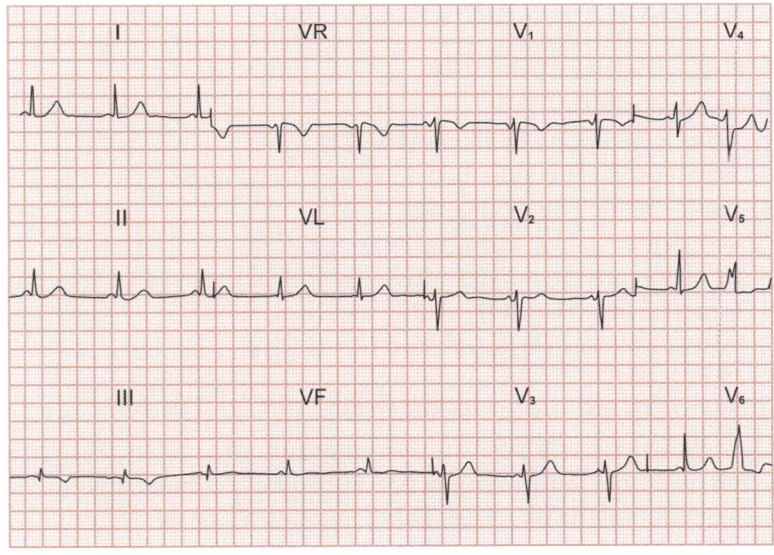

Fig. 62: Lown-Ganong-Levine syndrome. Short PR internal but normal QRS complex.

C. Varying
1. Wenckebach phenomenon **(Fig. 35)**
2. Wandering pacemaker **(Fig. 21)**

Q WAVE ABNORMALITIES

Pathological Q Wave
Q wave is wide (0.04 sec or more) and deep (more than 4 mm in depth):
1. In V_5, V_6, in LVH
2. In V_1, V_2 in RVH
3. In myocardial infarction—in leads II, III, aVF in: diaphragmatic infarction, and in aVL, V_5, V_6 in anterolateral infarction, and in V_1, V_2, V_3, V_4 in anteroseptal infarction. (Q waves exceed 25% of the height of the following R waves).
4. In pulmonary embolism, a Q wave may be seen in lead III, and a large S wave in lead I.
5. In presence of left bundle branch block (LBBB), Q waves appear in V_1, V_2, but q in V_5, V_6 signifies myocardial infarction.

QRS COMPLEX ABNORMALITIES

Duration and Amplitude
Prolonged QRS:
1. Ventricular premature beats **(Fig. 42)**
2. Intraventricular conduction defect (IVCD) **(Fig. 63)**
3. Bundle branch block **(Fig. 65)**
4. Ventricular tachycardia **(Fig. 30)**
5. Ectopic ventricular rhythm driven by artificial pacemaker **(Fig. 33)**
6. Hyperkalemia **(Fig. 60)**
7. WPW syndrome **(Figs. 64A and B)**

Intraventricular Conduction Defect (IVCD) (Fig. 63)
Here ventricles are activated from automatic cells within the ventricles either due to malfunction of all other potential rhythms or an irritability of the ventricles. Differentiation from supraventricular rhythm is from the duration of QRS complex (more than 0.10 sec).

Wolff-Parkinson-White (W-P-W) Syndrome (Pre-excitation Syndrome) (Figs. 64A and B)
Impulses originate in SA node and pre-excite peripheral conduction system and ventricle via accessory pathway which conducts the atrial impulse to the ventricular myocardium independent of the normal AV node. After delay at AV node impulses also arrive at ventricles

Method of Analysis of the Electrocardiogram

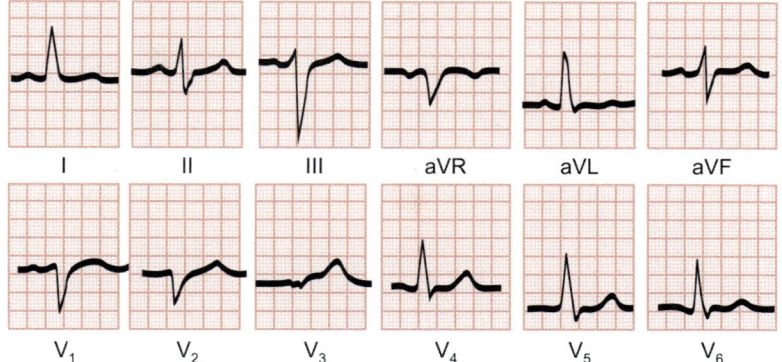

Fig. 63: Wide QRS complexes indicating intraventricular conduction defect.

via normal route to continue depolarization. Here the PR interval is abnormally short (<0.12 sec), and in addition a slurred upstroke (delta wave) is often seen in one or more leads. The WPW syndrome is due to route of conduction from atria to ventricles that bypasses the AV node. A small portion of ventriclular myocardium is thus excited early (Pre-excitation) producing the early slurred upstroke of the QRS complex. QRS is prolonged not because it lasted longer but because it started earlier as a result of pre-excitation.

In *type A WPW syndrome,* the accessory path is via bundle of Kent. There is an upright deflection in leads V1, V2 **(Fig. 64A)**. Lead V1 shows a tall, slurred R wave, lead V_6 a deep S wave. The ECG may be mistaken for RBBB or RV hypertrophy. In *type B,* impulses may pass via posterior accessory bundle. Lead V_1 shows a deep, wide S wave with a notch on the downstroke and leads V_5 and V_6 a tall slurred R wave. The ECG may be mistaken for LBBB or LV hypertrophy **(Fig. 64B)**.

Bundle Branch Block

Of the various forms of intraventricular block, bundle branch block is the most common.

Genesis of ECG pattern in bundle branch block. If one of the branches of the bundle of His is blocked by disease, the impulse will travel down the other ventricle first. Having activated this ventricle, the impulse will spread through the septum to the ventricle on the side of the block and in turn activate it. In other words, the ventricles will be activated one after the other instead of simultaneously. In BBB, since the impulse has to push its way through the thickness of the

Method of Analysis of the Electrocardiogram

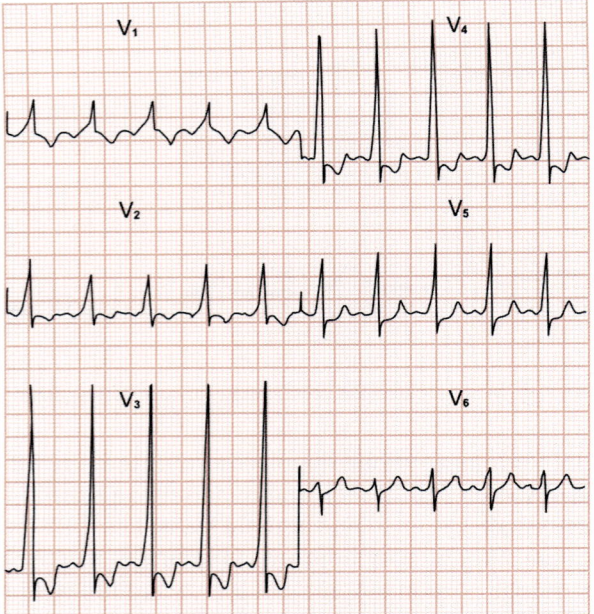

Fig. 64A: Type A WPW syndrome.

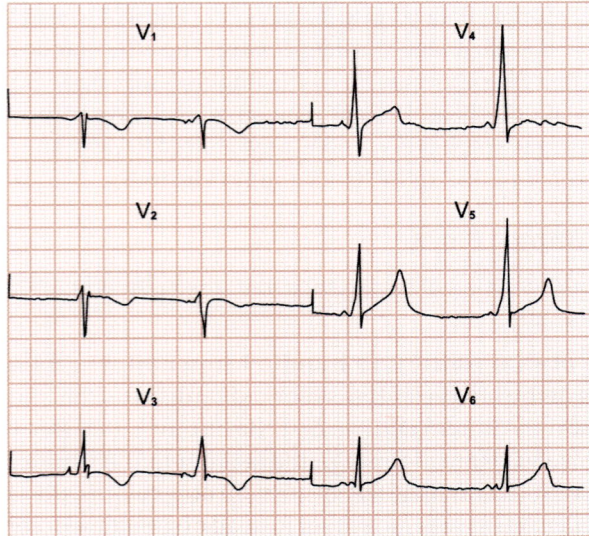

Fig. 64B: Type B WPW syndrome.

septum before the second ventricle can be activated, the QRS interval is prolonged to 0.12 second or more, it tends to be more prolonged in left than in right bundle branch block **(Fig. 65)**.

When the *left branch* is blocked **(Fig. 66)**, the impulse reaches the right ventricle punctually but it is late in activating the left ventricle. The intrinsicoid deflection over the right ventricle (V1) begins on time whereas over the left ventricle (V_6) the deflection is much delayed. When the *right branch* is blocked **(Fig. 67)**, the intrinsicoid deflection is on time over left ventricular leads but is late over the right ventricle. The QRS complex in right chest leads often becomes M shaped in RBBB, while S waves appear in left leads.

Types of bundle branch block

1. Right bundle branch block: The right bundle being long and slender is susceptible to damage.

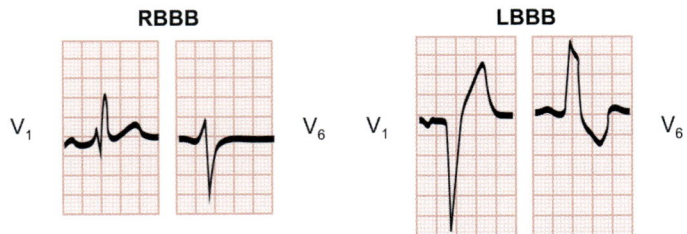

Fig. 65: Bundle branch block. The important leads to study in BBB are V_1 and V_6. (RBBB: right bundle branch block; LBBB: left bundle branch block)

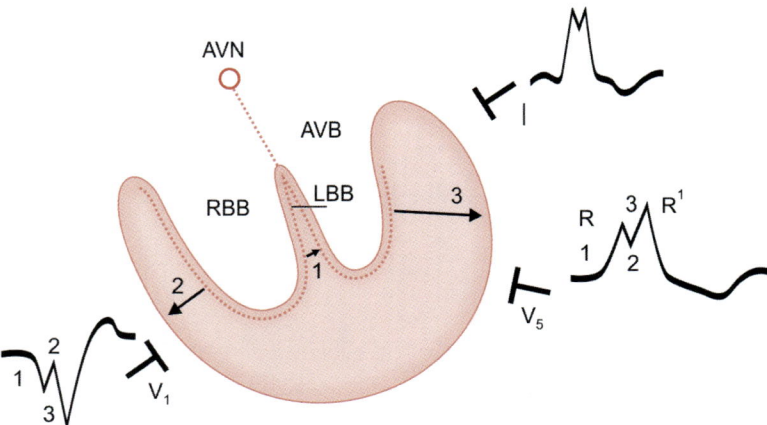

Fig. 66: Left bundle branch block. The genesis of M-shaped complex in V_5.

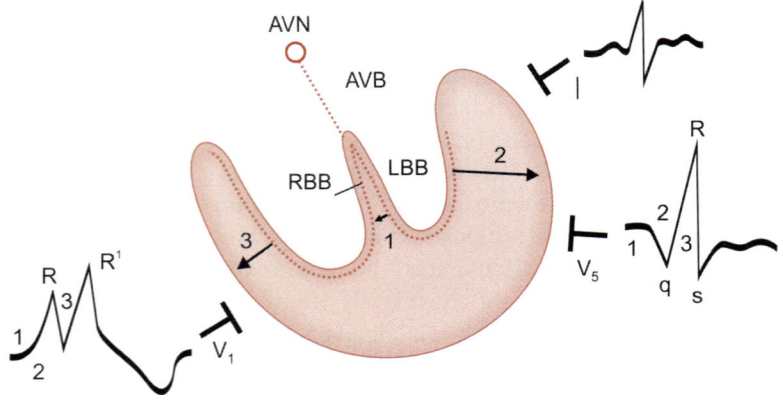

Fig. 67: Right bundle branch block— the genesis of RSR¹ pattern in V$_1$.

Complete RBBB—QRS more than 0.12 sec. with rsR pattern in right ventricular lead V$_1$ with negative T. Broad slurred S wave in I, V$_5$, V$_6$ **(Fig. 68)**.

Incomplete RBBB—QRS > 0.10 sec. but <0.12 sec.

2. **Left bundle branch block**

Complete LBBB—left ventricular leads V$_5$ and V$_6$ show broad, slurred and upright R wave with T in opposite direction **(Fig. 69)**. Similar pattern in I. Right ventricular leads show a deep negative deflection.

Incomplete LBBB—QRS >0.10 sec but <0.12 sec

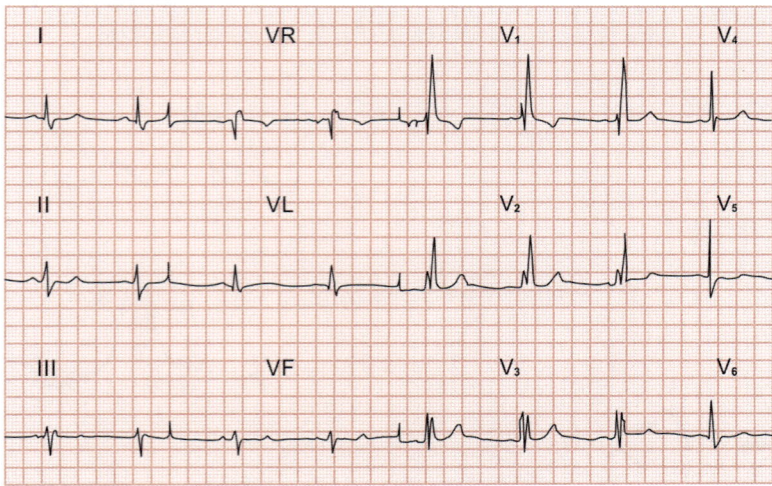

Fig. 68: Right bundle branch block. M-shaped complexes in right ventricular leads and delayed and slurred S waves in left ventricular leads.

Method of Analysis of the Electrocardiogram 49

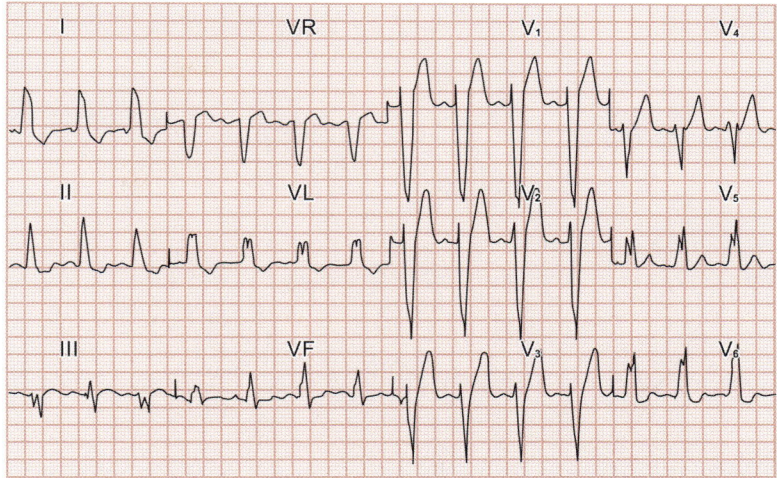

Fig. 69: Left bundle branch block. Note wide QRS with slurred R wave in V_{5-6}. Note absence of Q waves in lead I and V_{5-6}.

Block in the divisions of the left bundle
Both the divisions of the left bundle spread into fascicles which run through the walls of the left ventricle. The posterior division is thicker and shorter than the anterior division and has a double supply; hence, it is less prone to damage.

Left anterior hemiblock (LAHB) **(Fig. 70)**: Block of the anterior division of the left bundle results in:
1. Left axis deviation (because the terminal forces are redirected leftward and superiorly)
2. $Q_1 S_3$ pattern
3. Normal QRS duration
4. Small q wave in aVL

LAHB masks the signs of LVH or lateral wall ischemia in left precordial leads. It masks the signs of inferior wall infarct or ischemia in II, III, aVF.

Left posterior hemiblock (LPHB) **(Fig. 71)** *Results in:*
1. Right axis deviation (because the terminal forces are redirected rightward and inferiorly)
2. Normal QRS duration
3. $S_1 Q_3$ pattern

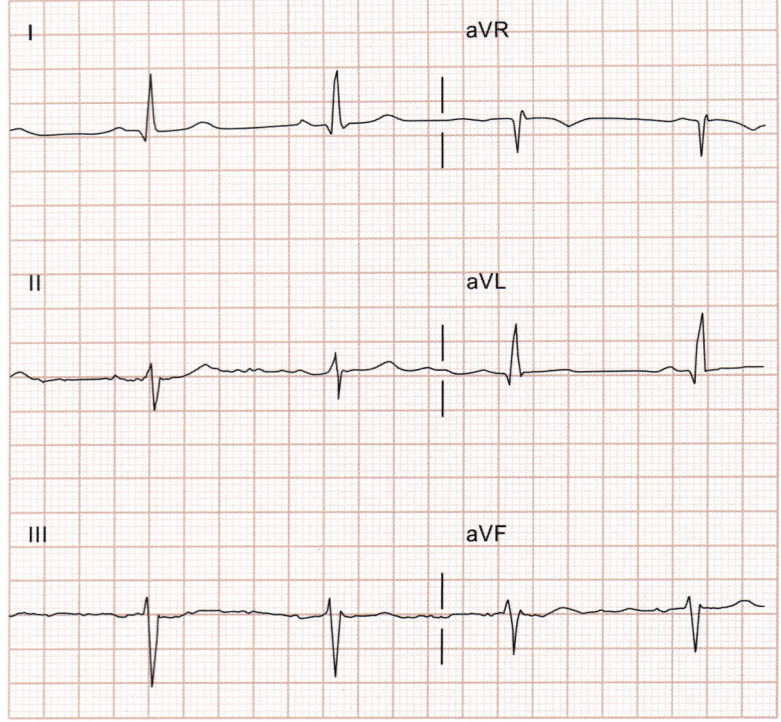

Fig. 70: Left anterior hemiblock.

Right ventricular hypertrophy and vertical heart should be excluded before diagnosis of LPHB.

Bilateral bundle branch block (BBBB)
a. *Bifascicular block:* The term fascicular block refers to a combination of blocks, e.g., hemiblock plus bundle branch block. Since, it is not generally possible to distiguish combination of anterior and posterior hemiblock from left bundle branch block, the term bifascicular block refers to (i) RBBB together with a block of either anterior (LAH) **(Fig. 72)** or (ii) posterior (LPH) **(Fig. 71)** division of left bundle branch. Posterior hemiblock in association with RBBB is considered dangerous since it is likely to progress to A-V blocks, including complete heart block.
b. *Trifascicular block* **(Fig. 73)**: Involvement of all the three fascicles, i.e., RBBB and both anterior and posterior divisions of the left

Method of Analysis of the Electrocardiogram

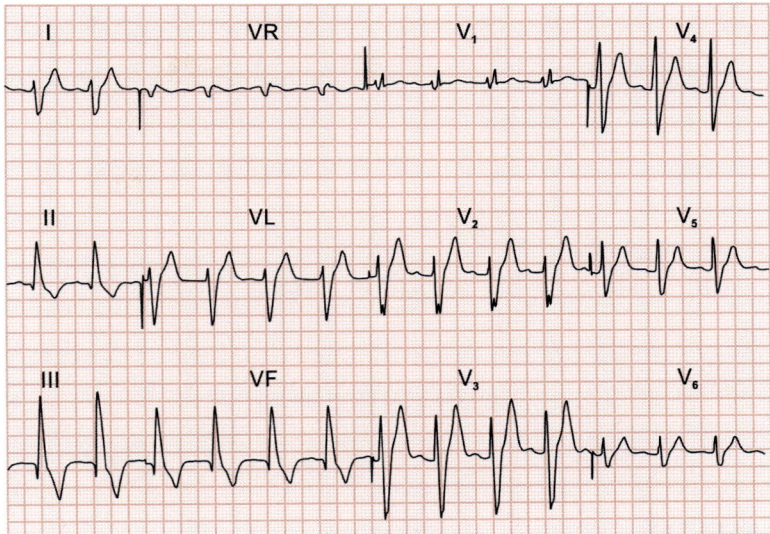

Fig. 71: Left posterior hemiblock.
Note associated RBBB with RAD.

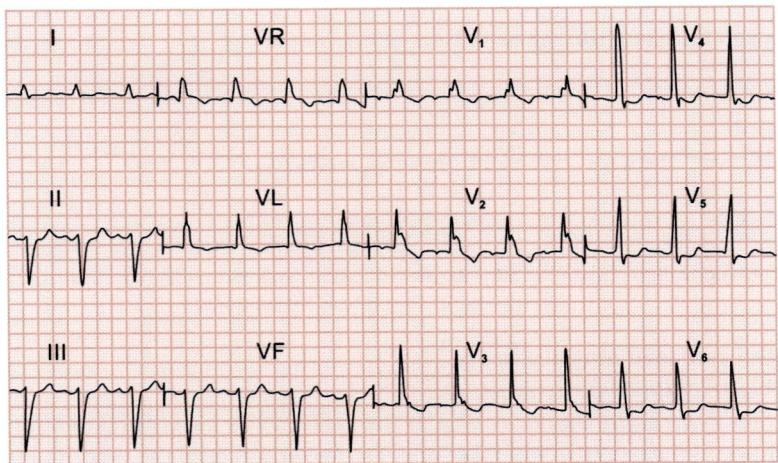

Fig. 72: RBBB with left anterior hemiblock (Bifascicular block).
RBBB pattern with LAD.

bundle, is a life threatening complication leading to complete heart block. It may be heralded by LBBB with prolonged PR interval or RBBB with prolonged PR interval.

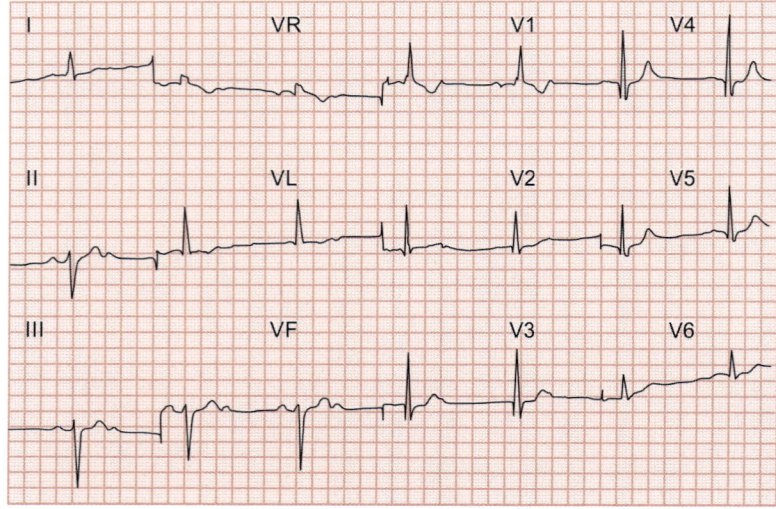

Fig. 73: Second degree (2:1) AV block with left anterior hemiblock and RBBB. (Trifascicular block).

Intermittent bundle branch block:
Bundle branch block may be permanent, or intermittent **(Fig. 74)** or even transient during exercise.

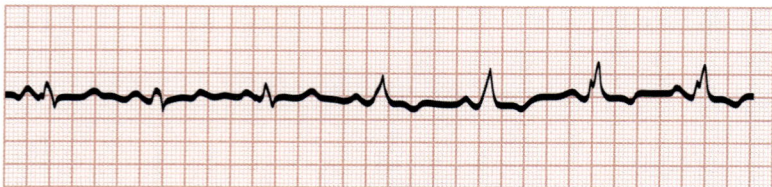

Fig. 74: Intermittent bundle branch block, last beats show bundle branch block pattern. P-P and R-R intervals are constant.

B. Increased amplitude:
Ventricular hypertrophy
Left ventricular hypertrophy: If the wall of the LV is thicker than normal the impulse will take longer to traverse it, and the ventricular activation time will be delayed over the leads facing LV, which will record tall R waves and correspondingly leads facing RV deep S waves **(Fig. 75)**.
Criteria for diagnosing LVH are:
1. R >25 mm, in V_5/V_6
2. S >25 mm, in V_1/V_2

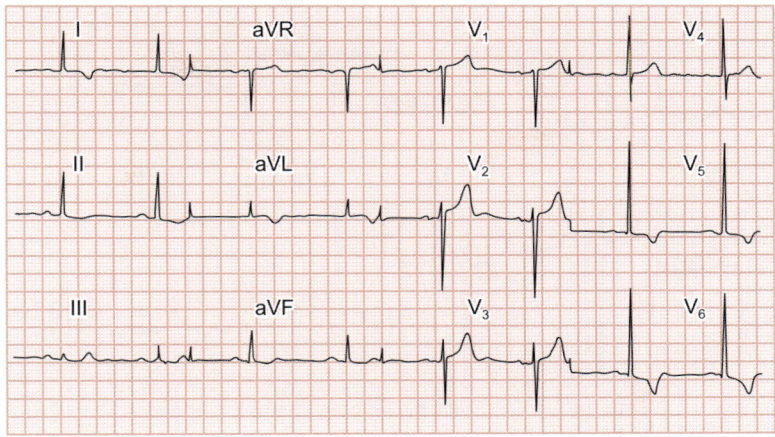

Fig. 75: Left ventricular hypertrophy. Tall R over left ventricle, deep S over right ventricle. Systolic overload.

3. R in V_5 or V_6 + S in V_1 >35 mm
4. R in I >14 mm.
5. R in a VL >11 mm.

LV systolic and diastolic overload: LVH may result from overload or strain either in systole (hypertension, aortic stenosis), or in diastole (AR, MR, PDA, VSD). In systolic overload pattern, T waves are inverted in V_5, V_6 **(Fig. 75)**, whereas in diastolic overload T waves are tall and upright in these leads **(Fig. 76)**.

Right ventricular hypertrophy: R waves in RV leads V_1 to V_4 will be tall and correspondingly deep S waves in LV leads V_5, V_6 **(Fig. 77)**. The RV occupies the whole of the anterior surface of the heart resulting in clockwise rotation.

Criteria for diagnosing RVH are:
1. R in V_1 > S in V_1
2. R in V_1 + S in V_5 or V_6 >10 mm
3. R in V_1 >1 mm
4. S m V_5 >7 mm
5. qR pattern in V_1

Biventricular hypertrophy
At times, the potentials from the two hypertrophied ventricles cancel each other so that the cardiogram may appear normal. Biventricular hypertrophy may be diagnosed if—precordial leads show RVH in right ventricular leads and LVH in left ventricular leads **(Fig. 78)**.

Method of Analysis of the Electrocardiogram

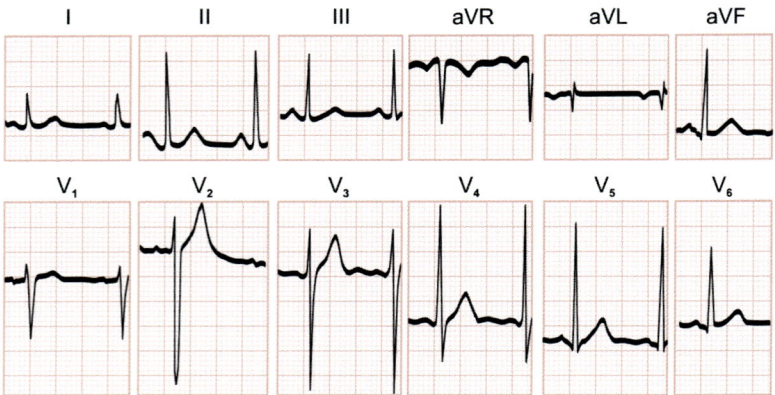

Fig. 76: Left ventricular hypertrophy. Diastolic overload.

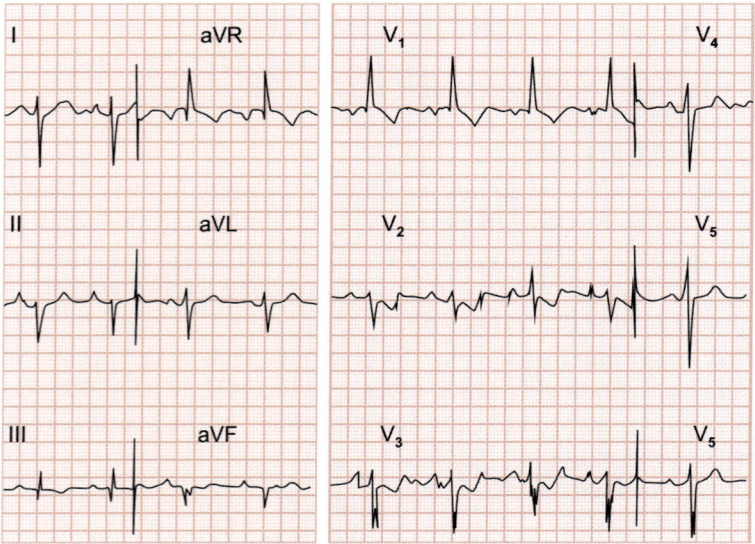

Fig. 77: Right ventricular hypertrophy tall R waves in V_1.

■ ST SEGMENT ABNORMALITIES

A. Depressed

1. **Digitalis effect:** ST segment is depressed and sagging with a gradual downward slope and ending in a terminal rise to isoelectric level **(Fig. 79)**. It has hence been compared to the mirror-image of a

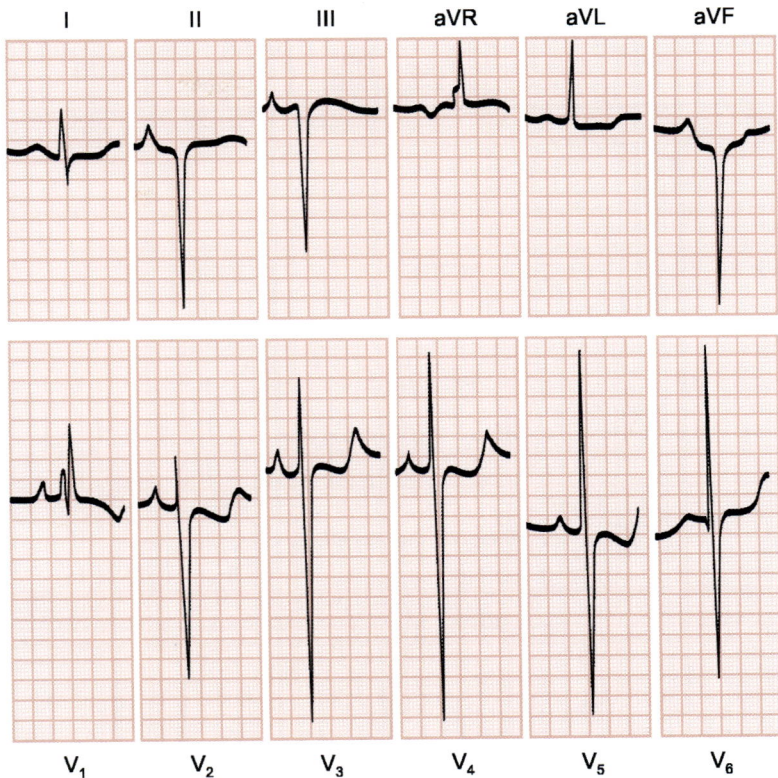

Fig. 78: Biventricular hypertrophy. Evidence of LVH in left ventricular leads and RVH in right ventricular leads.

correction mark or hockey stick pattern. The effect is best seen in leads with tallest R waves.
2. **LV strain:** ST depressed and convex upwards with asymmetrical T wave inversion in left precordial leads **(Fig. 80).**
3. **RV strain:** Same as LV strain but in right ventricular leads **(Fig. 81).**
4. **Myocardial ischemia:** Ischemic ST segment shows greater than 1 mm ST depression in more than two leads, with horizontal (flat) or down-sloping ST configuration **(Fig. 82).**

B. Elevated

1. **Pericarditis:** The epicardial surface of the heart is inflamed or injured in pericarditis. This is reflected in raised ST segments in

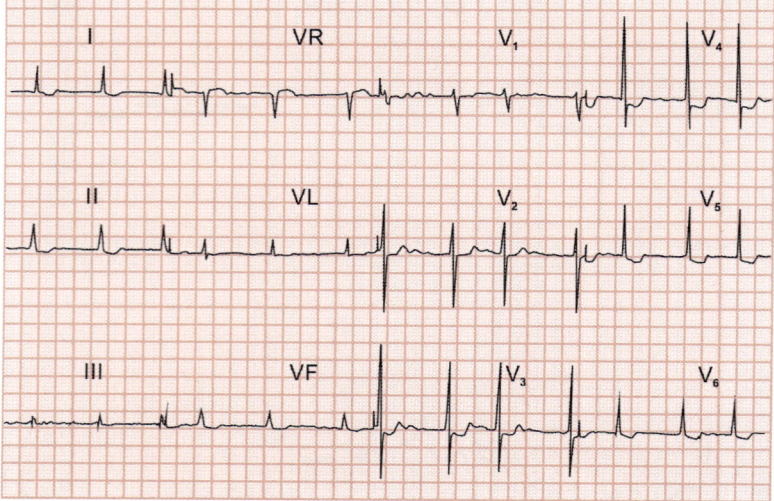

Fig. 79: Digitalis effect.

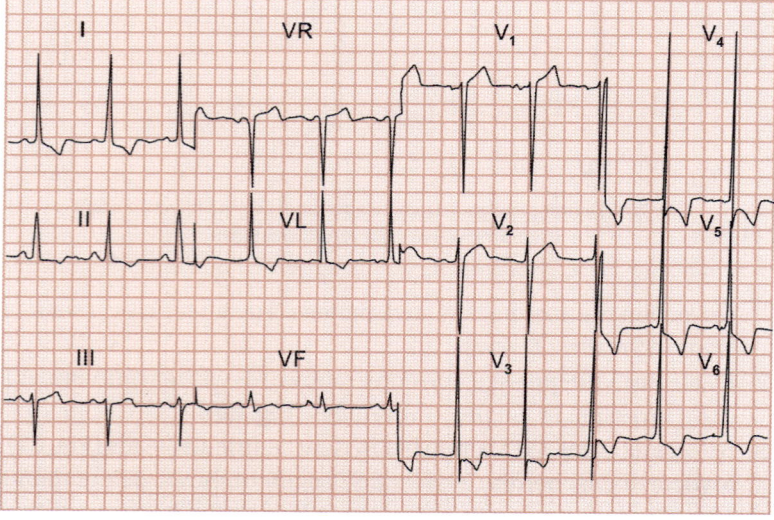

Fig. 80: Left ventricular hypertrophy with strain.

epicardial leads overlying the affected zone. Since, pericarditis is a diffuse process the changes are seen in all leads **(Fig. 83).**

2. **Myocardial infarction:** The most characteristic finding in acute myocardial infarction is elevation of the ST segment in leads

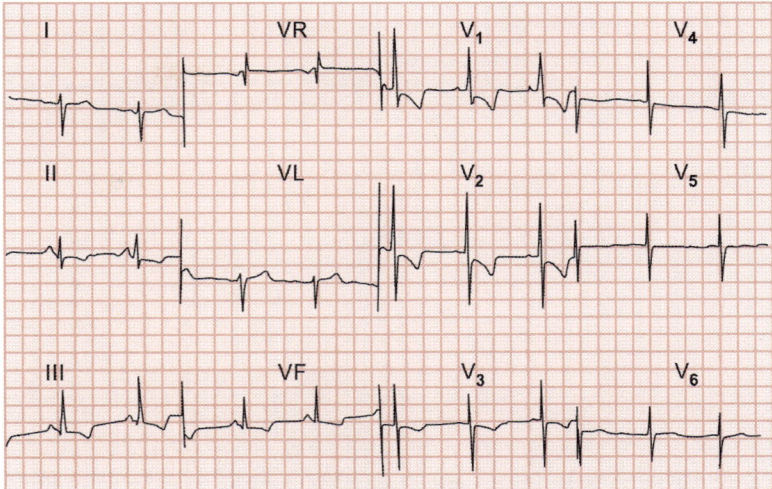

Fig. 81: Right ventricular hypertrophy with strain.

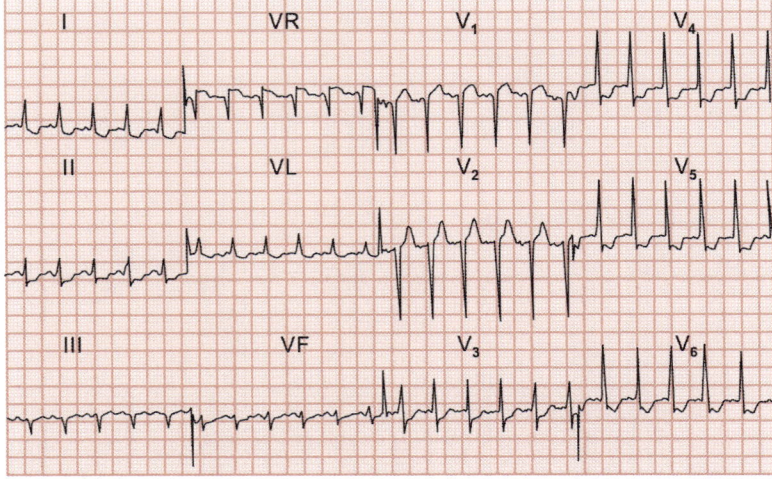

Fig. 82: Severe myocardial ischemia. Q waves are absent and several of the limb and precordial leads show ST depression.

recorded over the area involved **(Fig. 84)**. There may be reciprocal ST depression in leads recorded over the opposite part of the heart.

3. **Normal:** ST segment is sometimes normally elevated not more than 1 mm in standard leads and even 2 mm in some of the chest leads.

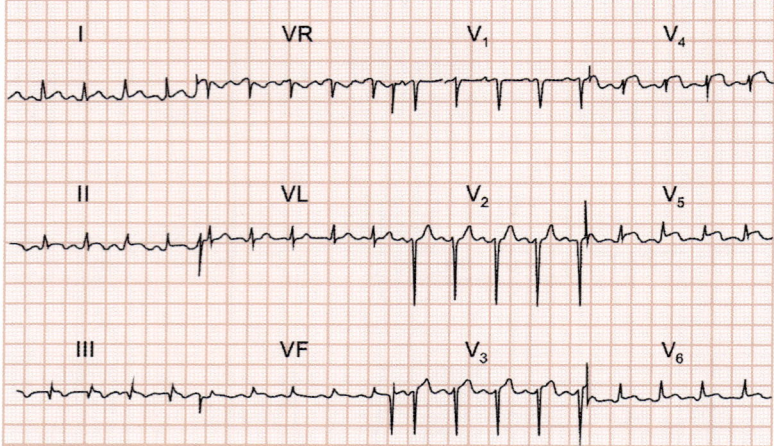

Fig. 83: Acute pericarditis. Raised ST segments in all leads facing the injured surface except aVR which faces the cavity of the heart (uninjured surface). Note that the ST segment concavity is upward ("saddle-back" appearance).

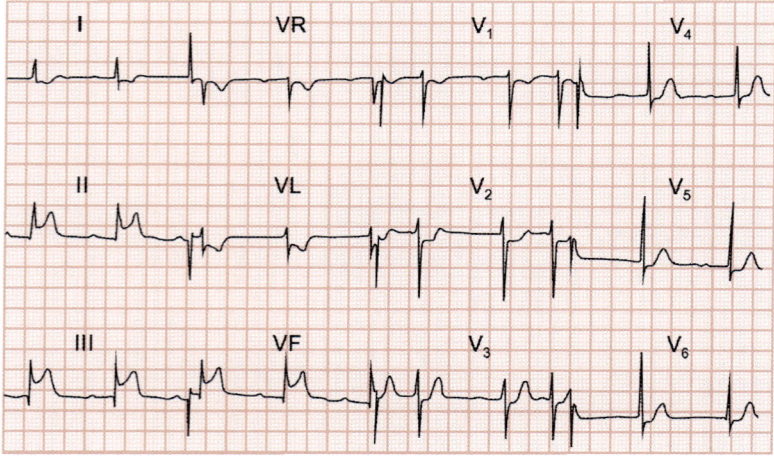

Fig. 84: Acute inferior myocardial infarction.

When a raised ST segment follows a S wave, it is called 'high take-off' ST segment. This is a normal variant **(Fig. 85)**.

4. **Early repolarization (Fig. 86)**: ST segment elevation up to 4 mm in left precordial leads with upright T waves can be seen in normal individuals. This results from early repolarization which

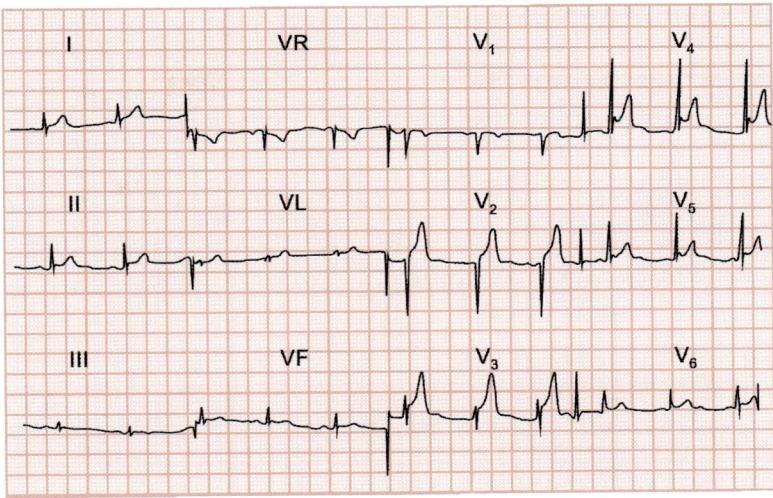

Fig. 85: High take-off ST segment.

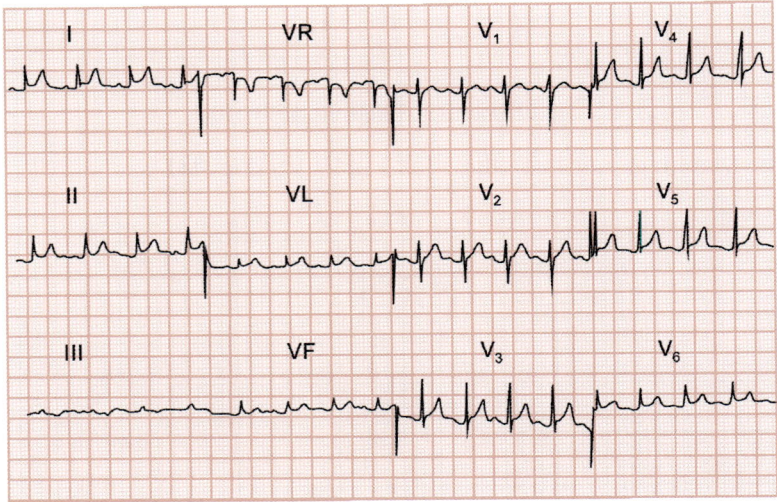

Fig. 86: ECG in early repolarization showing ST elevation with concavity upward. A notch at the end of R wave, is seen in some leads.

occurs before depolarization is completed in other areas of the myocardium. The elevated ST segment shows an upward concavity. Also a notch may be present at the end of R wave.

T WAVE ABNORMALITIES

A. Increased Amplitude

1. Normal (in V_2 to V_5) **(Fig. 87)**

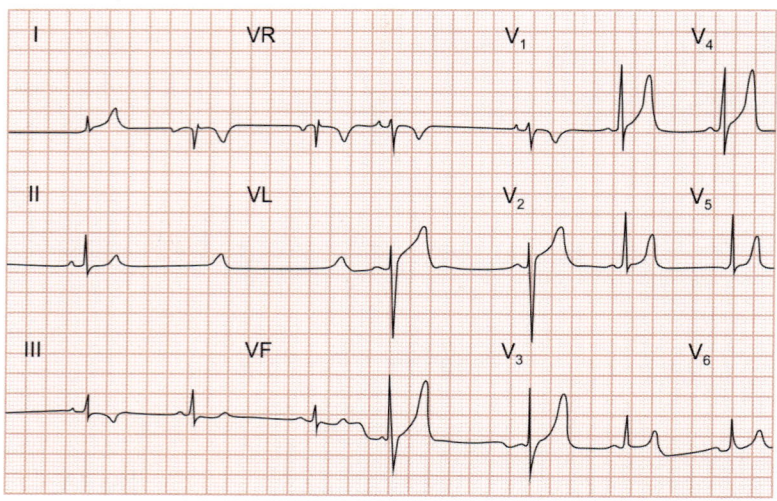

Fig. 87: Normal ECG. Note the tall T Waves.

2. Diaphragmatic infarction (Tall T in V_1, V_2) **(Fig. 88)**

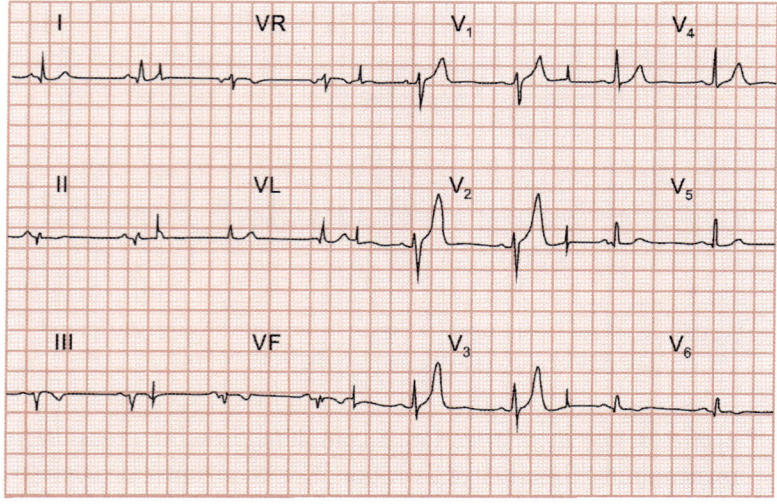

Fig. 88: Inferior myocardial infarction.

3. True posterior infarct
4. Myocardial ischemia without infarction
5. Hyperkalemia **(Fig. 89)**
6. Cerebrovascular events.

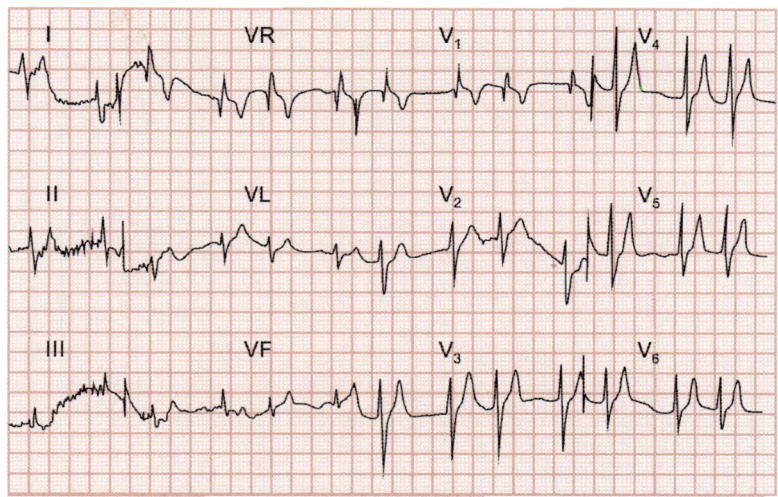

Fig. 89: Hyperkalemia. Tall peaked T waves usually greatest in precordial leads are earliest change. Atrial standstill may develop as serum potassium increases.

B. Low or Flat

1. Myocardial ischemia or infarction
2. Digitalis effect
3. Hypothyroidism
4. Constrictive pericarditis
5. Myocarditis
6. Hypokalemia

C. Inverted

1. Premature beats
2. Bundle branch block
3. Myocardial ischemia or infarction
4. Pericarditis
5. Ventricular strain
6. Myocarditis
7. Cardiomyopathy **(Fig. 90)**
8. Pulmonary embolism

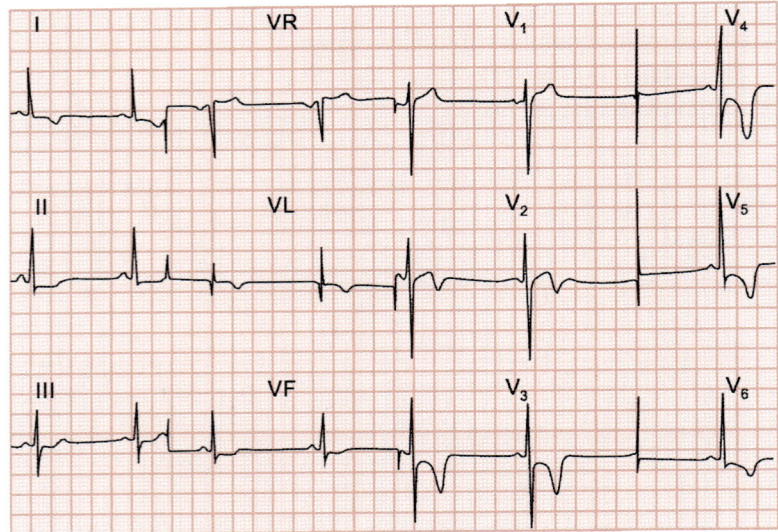

Fig. 90: T wave inversion in hypertrophic cardiomyopathy.

QT INTERVAL ABNORMALITIES

Q-TC interval is the QT interval corrected for heart rate.

$$Q\text{-}TC = \sqrt{\frac{Q\text{-}T \text{ interval}}{RR \text{ interval}}}$$ Normally less than 0.44 sec.

Prolonged
1. Diffuse myocardial disease
2. Myocardial infarction
3. Hypocalcemia
4. Class IA, IC and III antiarrhythmic agents
5. Rheumatic fever and other causes of acute myocarditis
6. Head injury or cerebrovascular accident
7. Hypothermia
8. Congenital long QT syndrome **(Fig. 91)**
9. Hypothyroidism

Shortened
1. Digitalis effect

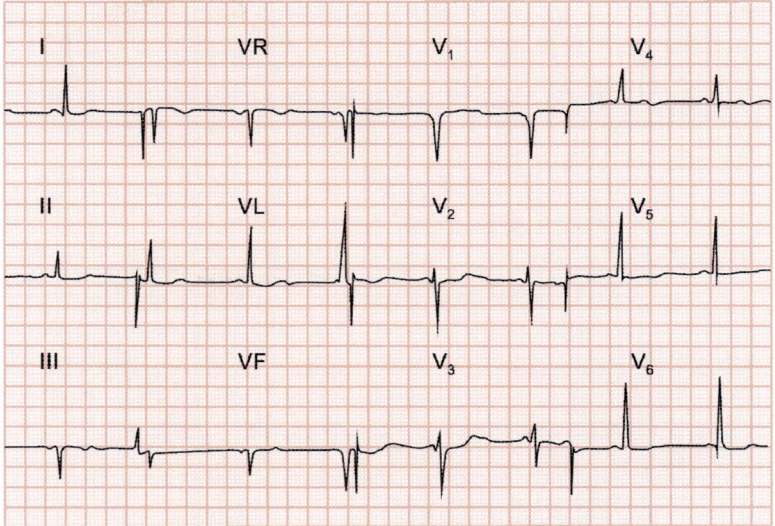

Fig. 91: Congenital long QT syndrome. QTC = 0.60 sec.

2. Hypercalcemia
3. Hyperkalemia

■ U WAVE ABNORMALITIES

- **Prominent**: Hypokalemia **(Fig. 92)**. Digoxin toxicity, hypercalcemia.
- **Inverted**: Ischemic or hypertensive heart disease.

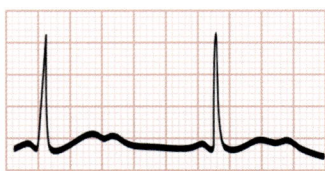

Fig. 92: Prominent 'U waves'.

■ J WAVE

The junction of QRS complex and ST segment is referred to as the J segment. In *hypothermia,* the J wave appears as a hump-like wave usually superimposed on the distal limb of QRS complex **(Fig. 93)**.

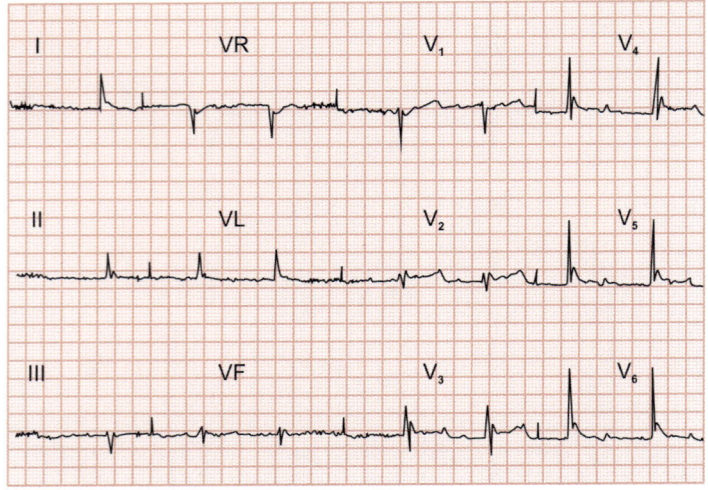

Fig. 93: Electrocardiogram showing J waves in a hypothermic patient.

CHAPTER 4

Ischemic Heart Disease

■ MYOCARDIAL INFARCTION (MI)

ECG Changes in ST Segment Elevation MI (STEMI)

The electrocardiogram is of great value in the diagnosis of myocardial infarction. When occlusion of the coronary blood supply occurs, that portion of the myocardium progresses through three stages of increasing damage towards infarction. These could be recorded if a precordial lead is placed directly over the site affected:
1. Ischemia with inversion of T wave
2. Injury with elevation of ST segment
3. Infarction or muscle death, recognized by appearance of Q wave and decrease in amplitude or disappearance of R wave **(Fig. 94).**

These changes are registered in leads which face the area of damage. Opposite or reciprocal changes (no Q wave, depressed ST and tall upright T) are recorded in leads facing the diametrically opposed site of infarction.

Genesis of the Q Wave

If the area of infarction extends from endocardial to epicardial surface of the myocardium (transmural infarct), it produces an 'electrical hole' between the exploring electrode and the ventricular cavity. Since, dead tissue is capable of conduction, the normal negative cavity potential will be recorded by an overlying electrode as QS deflection and by a neighboring electrode as an abnormal Q wave. The depth of Q will depend on the location of the exploring electrode in relation to the area of infarction.

Ischemic Heart Disease

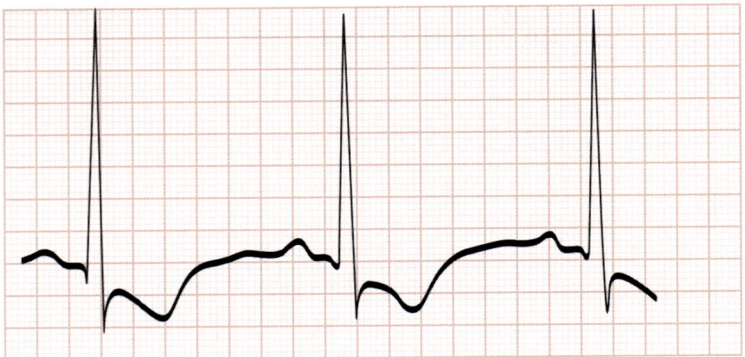

Zone of myocardial ischemia

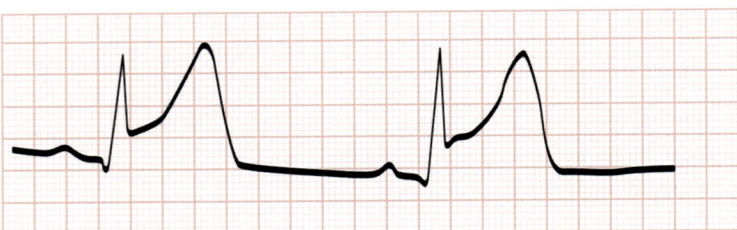

Zone of injury

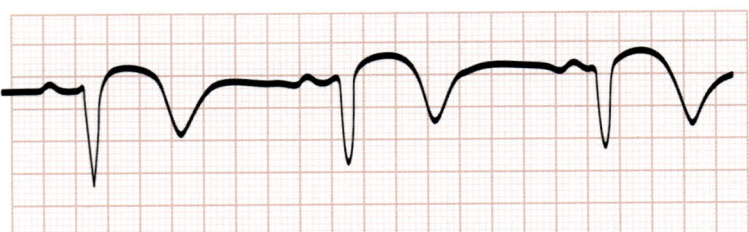

Zone of infarction

Fig. 94: The ECG patterns of ischemia, injury and infarction.

This phenomenon can also be interpreted in the sense that there is a loss of electrical forces directed towards the electrode placed over the necrotic or infarcted area, in other words the electrical forces tend to move away from the area, thus resulting in a negative deflection (Q or QS).

Ischemic Heart Disease

Location of areas of myocardial infarction, and their relation to ECG leads:

ST Elevation	Area of Infarction
V_1–V_2	Septal
V_3–V_4	Anterior
V_1 to V_4	Anteroseptal
I, aVL, V_5, V_6	Lateral
I, aVL, V_3 to V_6	Anterolateral
I, aVL, V_1 to V_6	Extensive anterior
II, III, aVF	Inferior
V_4R, V_5R, V_6R	Right ventricular
II, III, aVF, V_5, V_6	Inferolateral

- **Anterior infarction:** The anterior surface of the left ventricle usually faces aVL (hence lead I) and the precordial leads. Anterior infarction can be subdivided into:
    - *Antero-lateral:* Abnormal Q waves in I, aVL, and V_3 to V_6 **(Fig. 95)**. In lateral infarction changes may be seen only in aVL **(Fig. 96)**.
    - *Anteroseptal:* Characteristic changes in V_1, V_2, V_3 and V_4 **(Fig. 97)**.
    - *Extensive anterior*: Q, ST and T changes in I, aVL and all precordial leads from V_1 to V_6 **(Fig. 98)**.
- **Inferior infarction**: The inferior or diaphragmatic surface of the heart usually faces lead aVF (hence leads II and III) and the epigastric lead Ve. Changes of infarction are best seen in II, III, aVF and Ve **(Fig. 99)** and may not appear at all in the chest leads.
    - *Inferolateral:* It is shown in V_5 and V_6 and inferior leads.
- **Posterior infarction:** Normally, the electrical forces of the anterior ventricular wall are counteracted by forces of the posterior ventricular wall resulting in a small force anteriorly in the form of r wave in V_1, V_2. In true posterior infarction, the posterior force is lost and since the anterior force is no longer opposed, a large force in the form of R waves results anteriorly. Diagnosis is made from tall R waves in V_1, V_2 **(Fig. 100)** and peaked upright T waves.

Ischemic Heart Disease

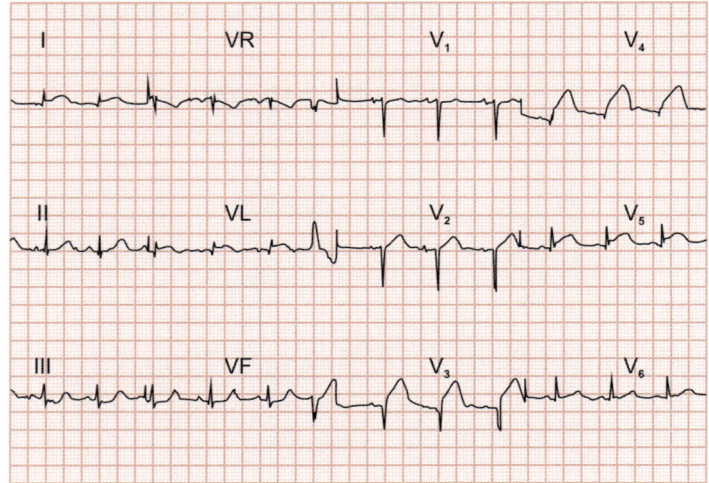

Fig. 95: Acute anterolateral infarction.

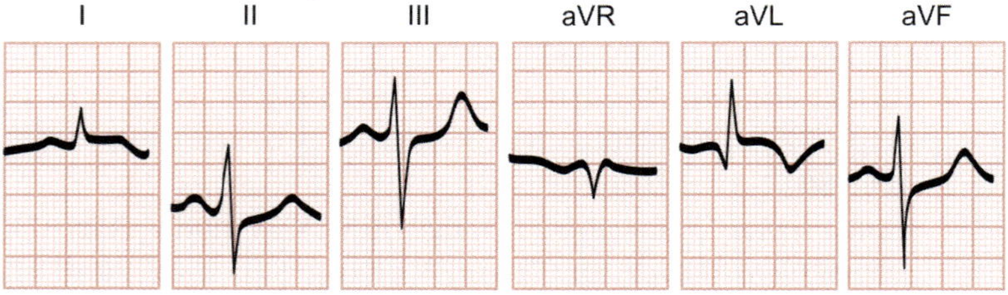

Fig. 96: Lateral infarction (Lead aVL).

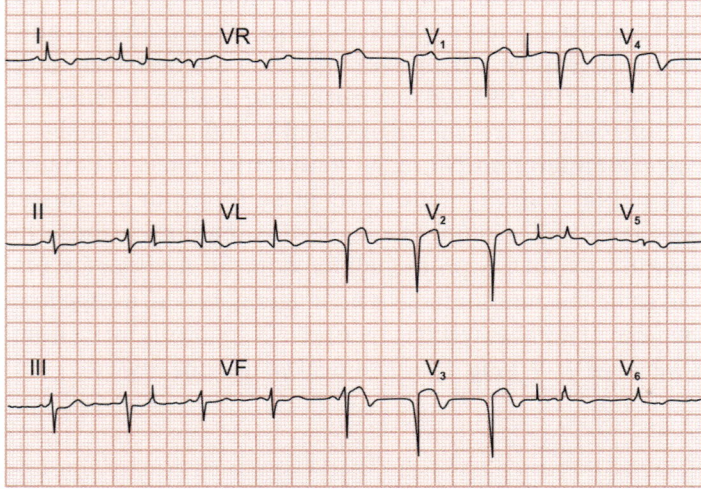

Fig. 97: Anteroseptal MI.

Ischemic Heart Disease 69

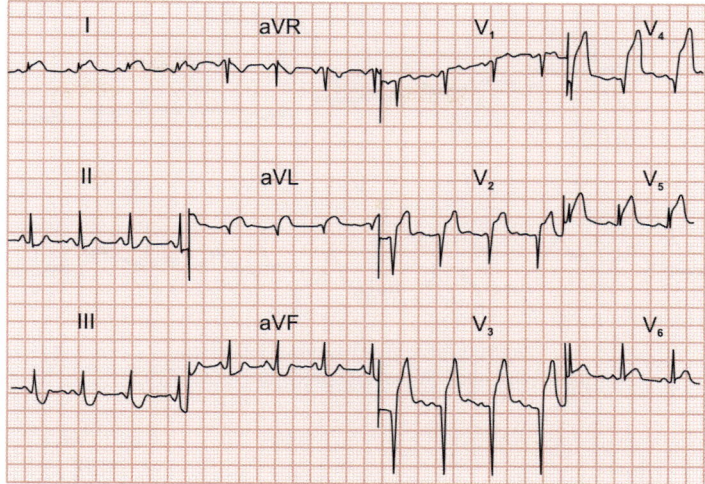

Fig. 98: Acute extensive anterior infarction.

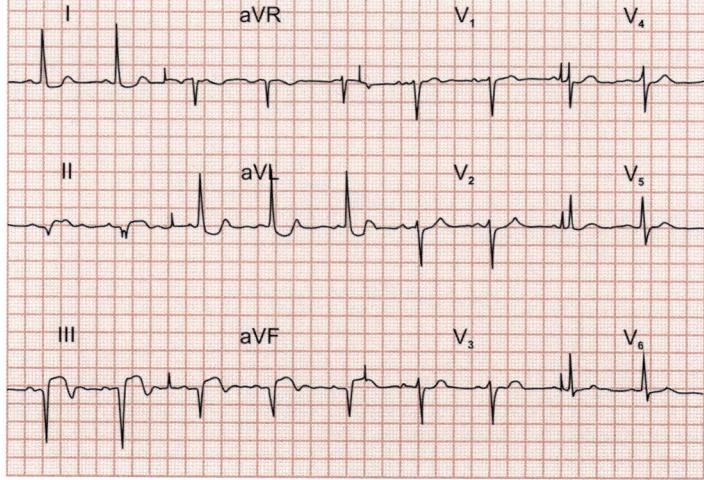

Fig. 99: Acute inferior infarction.

ECG Changes in Non-ST Segment Elevation MI (NSTEMI)

There is depression of ST with T wave inversion in several of the limb and precordial leads **(Fig. 101)**. There is no Q wave because the infarct

Ischemic Heart Disease

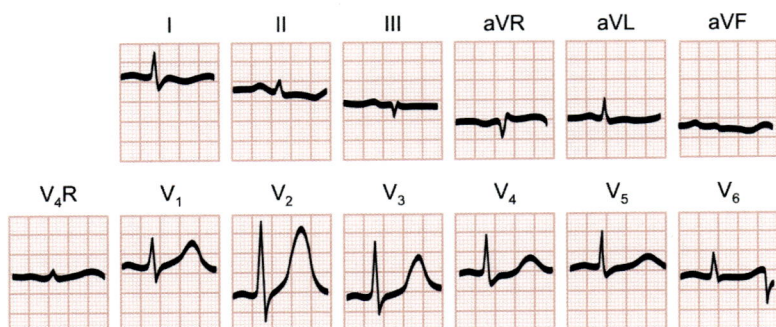

Fig. 100: Posterior myocardial infarction. Note tall R and T in the right precordial leads (V_1, V_2).

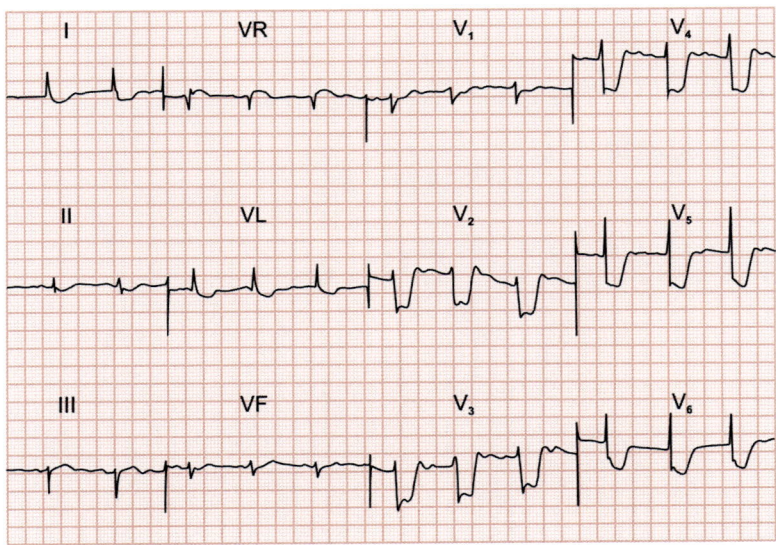

Fig. 101: Acute non-Q wave (non-ST elevation) infarction. From a patient with the clinical picture of infarction; note widespread ST-T depression in limb and chest leads, but no associated Q waves.

lies on the endocardial portion of the myocardium, the epicardial region is not infarcted.

- **Evolution of infarction:** The various phases in the evolution of a myocardial infarct can be demonstrated in serial cardiograms taken over a period of time. The changes may be divided into four stages **(Fig. 102)**:

Ischemic Heart Disease

- *Stage 1:* Acute phase as a rule in the first few hours. Abnormal Q waves, raised ST segments.
- *Stage 2:* Gradual return of elevated ST segments to base line, T begins to become inverted.
- *Stage 3:* Q waves persist, ST isoelectric, T waves symmetrically and deeply inverted (arrow head inversion).
- *Stage 4:* The residual or stabilized phase, where T waves gradually become shallower and return to normal. The only evidence that may remain of a previous infarction may be a pathological Q wave, but sometimes with a good collateral circulation the necrotic area shrinks to such small dimensions that Q waves may also disappear and no residual evidence of infarction is left.

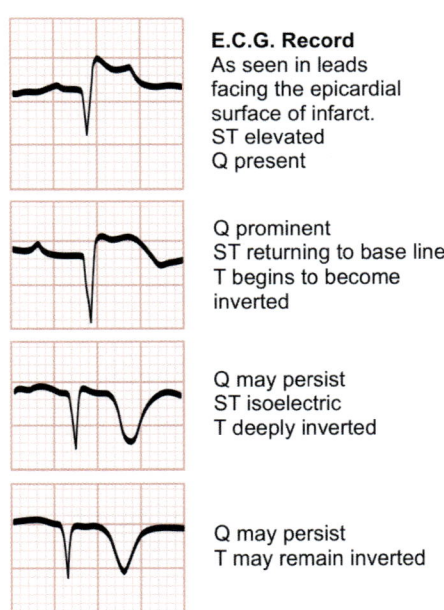

E.C.G. Record
As seen in leads facing the epicardial surface of infarct.
ST elevated
Q present

Q prominent
ST returning to base line.
T begins to become inverted

Q may persist
ST isoelectric
T deeply inverted

Q may persist
T may remain inverted

Fig. 102: Evolutionary changes of myocardial infarction.

Significance of persistent changes:
1. Persistent ST segment changes suggest possibility of ventricular aneurysm.
2. Sometimes, persistent changes are due to replacement of muscle by fibrous tissue, resulting in low voltage of QRS complexes.

Causes of absence of significant ECG changes:
1. Small area of infarction
2. Simultaneous infarcts, one neutralizing the pattern of the other
3. Anterior infarction with LBBB (but 'q' in V_5, V_6)

■ MYOCARDIAL ISCHEMIA WITHOUT INFARCTION

Electrocardiographic studies of patients suffering from chronic angina pectoris or coronary artery disease can be made in the following situations: (1) At rest in the interval between episodes of anginal pain. (2) During an anginal attack. (3) During or after a period of stress or effort tests.

ECG at Rest

A patient suffering from angina pectoris may have a normal cardiogram or the ECG may show changes suggestive of myocardial ischemia **(Fig. 103)**. The contour abnormality of ST consists of a change from the normal ST segment to a concave contour, to one having a horizontal course or downslope of ST segment. A further change is depression of ST below the isoelectric line, or by sagging of ST segment, or inversion of T wave.

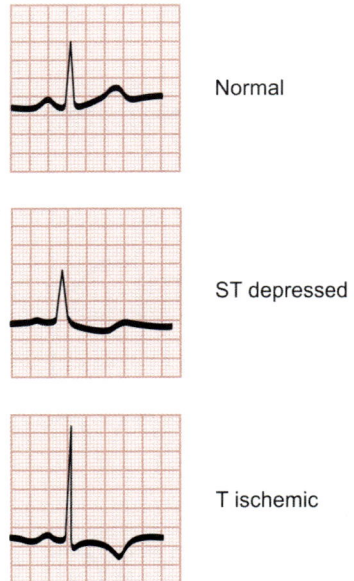

Fig. 103: Changes in ST segments and T waves in ischemic heart disease.

ECG During Anginal Attack

Theoretically, the most reliable information regarding the nature of ECG changes resulting from or associated with angina can be obtained during a spontaneous episode of angina. ECG will show transitory ischemic ST-T changes **(Fig. 104)**.

Ischemic Heart Disease

No Pain

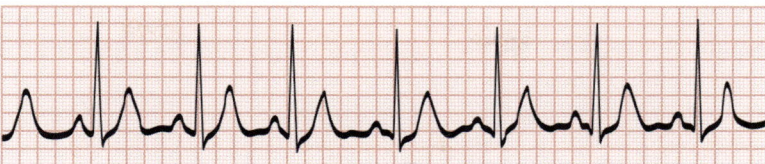

Chest Pain

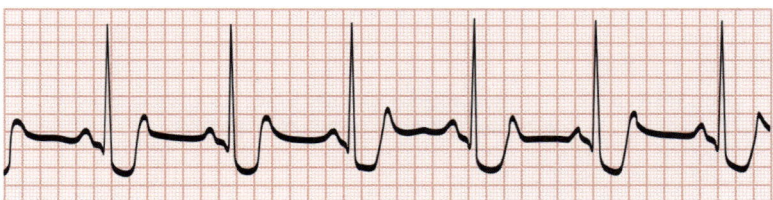

Fig. 104: ECG tracing before onset of chest pain and during pain when there is marked ST segment depression.

Prinzmetal's (Variant) Angina

Angina at rest caused by coronary artery spasm may be accompanied by ST elevation instead of depression. The ECG appears as in acute ST elevation myocardial infarction (STEMI) **(Fig. 105A)**, but ST elevation returns to normal when angina subsides **(Fig. 105B)**.

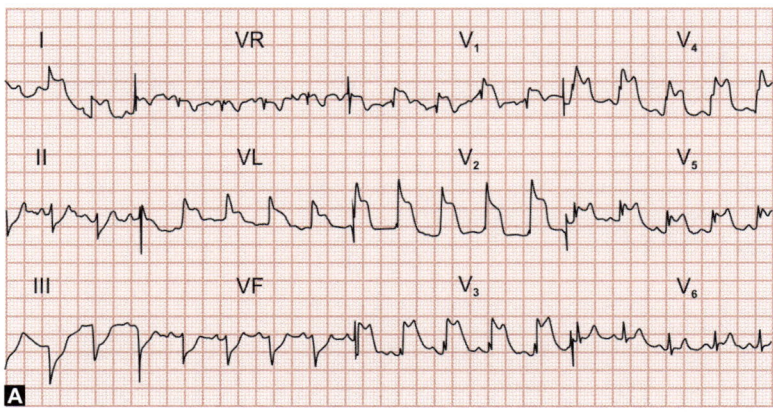

Ischemic Heart Disease

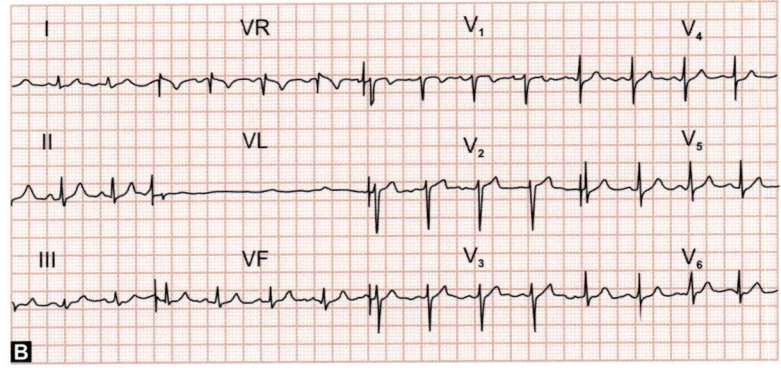

Figs. 105A and B: Prinzmetal's angina—elevated ST segment during angina in V_1 to V_5, returning to normal when angina settles.

The Brugada Syndrome

A genetic abnormality of sodium transport in the myocardium, predisposes to ventricular tachycardia and fibrillation.

The ECG resembles a right bundle branch block (RBBB) pattern in V_1 and V_2, with an elevated ST segment which is downward-sloping. However, there is no prominent S wave in V_6 as in RBBB **(Fig. 106)**.

The ECG changes are not constant, and the patient may have a normal ECG on another tracing.

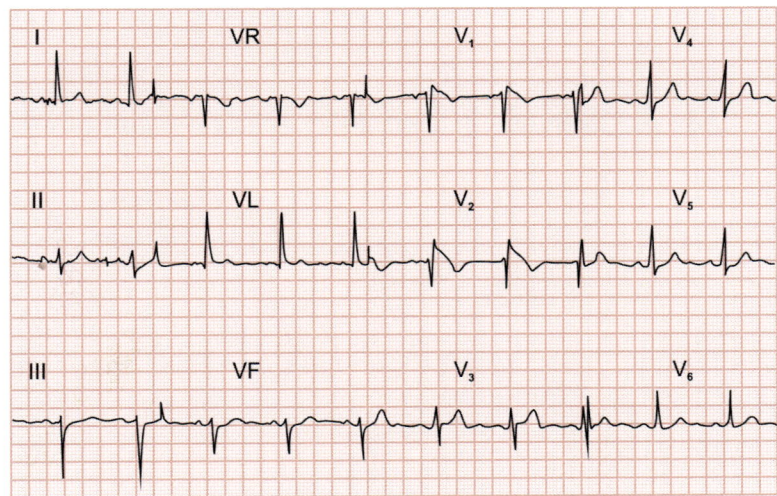

Fig. 106: Brugada syndrome. ST segment elevated in V_1 and V_2.